FEEL
GREAT
LOSE
WEIGHT

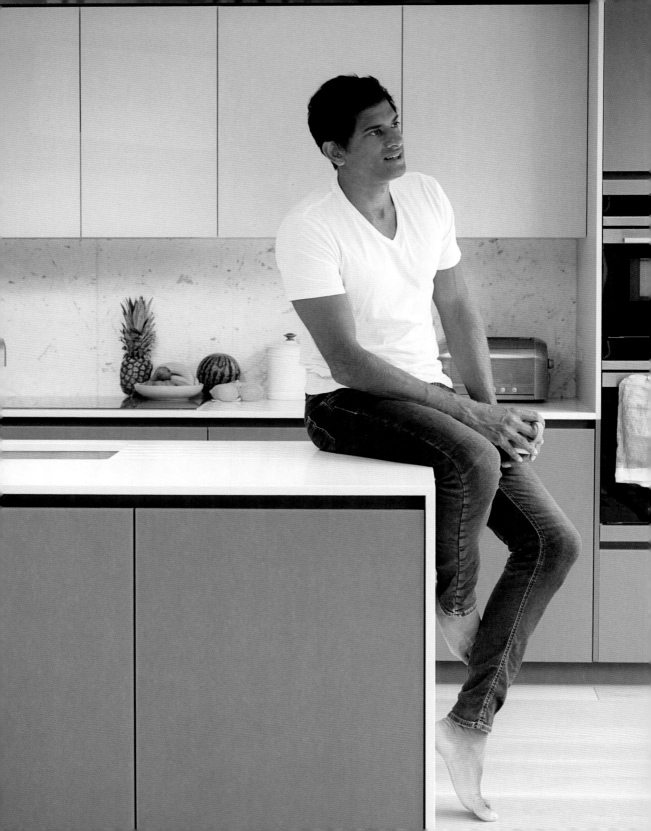

DR. RANGAN CHATTERJEE

FEEL GREAT LOSE WEIGHT

Long-term, simple habits for lasting and sustainable weight loss

PHOTOGRAPHY BY CLARE WINFIELD

BenBella Books, Inc.
Dallas, TX

This book is for informational purposes only. It is not intended to serve as a substitute for professional medical advice. The author and publisher specifically disclaim any and all liability arising directly or indirectly from the use of any information contained in this book. A health care professional should be consulted regarding your specific medical situation.

BenBella

BenBella Books, Inc.
10440 N. Central Expressway
Suite 800
Dallas, TX 75231
www.benbellabooks.com
Send feedback to feedback@benbellabooks.com

BenBella is a federally registered trademark.

Printed in the United States of America
10 9 8 7 6 5 4 3 2 1

Library of Congress Cataloging-in-Publication Data is available upon request.
LCCN: 2020049113
ISBN 9781953295057 (trade paperback)
ISBN 9781953295194 (ebook)

Cover design by Sarah Avinger
Cover photo © Shutterstock / Alex Staroseltsev

Originally published by Penguin Random House UK

Distributed to the trade by Two Rivers Distribution, an Ingram brand
www.tworiversdistribution.com

Special discounts for bulk sales are available.
Please contact bulkorders@benbellabooks.com

FOR JAINAM AND ANOUSHKA

I HOPE THIS BOOK CONTRIBUTES
TO A MORE COMPASSIONATE
WORLD FOR YOU TO GROW UP AND
THRIVE IN

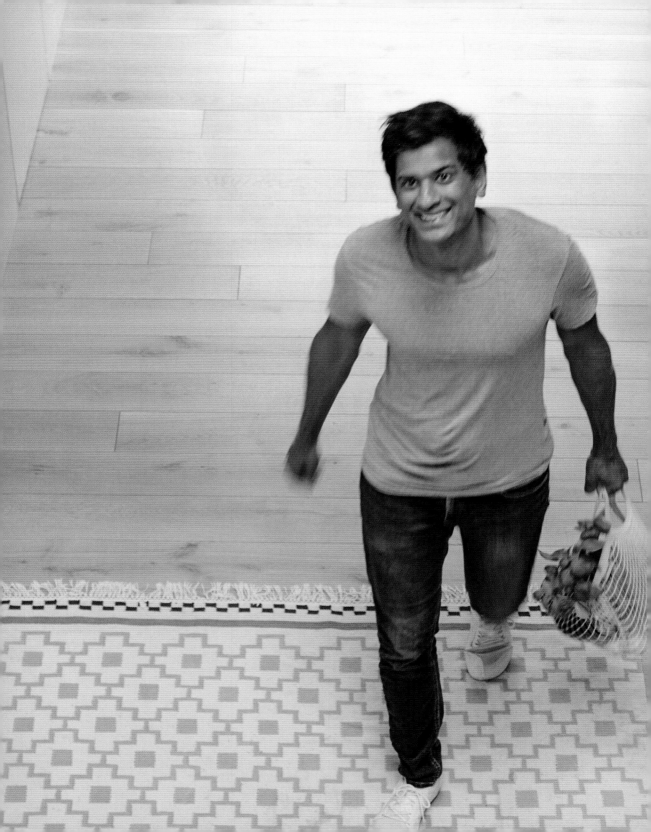

CONTENTS

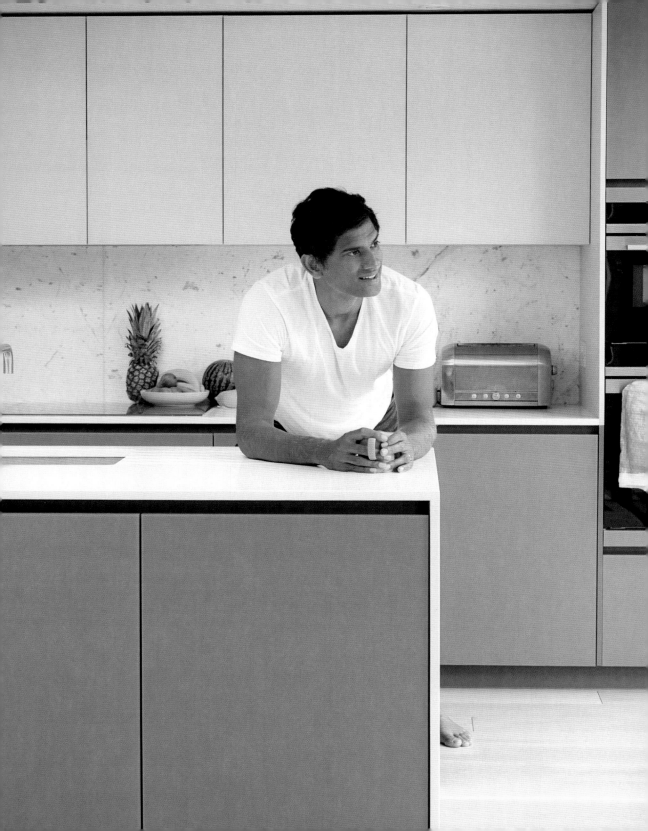

YOU HAVE ENTERED A NO-BLAME ZONE

It's time to stop feeling bad about yourself. It's time to stop beating yourself up. It's time to stop blaming yourself for all the struggles you might have had in the past about your weight. It's time to get smart about how to solve them. It's time for a new approach—one that's scientifically sound, doesn't make you feel tired or annoyed or hungry—and one that actually works.

If you're someone who struggles with maintaining a healthy weight and tends to judge yourself negatively, I have something important to tell you. It honestly can't wait a moment longer. It's harder for you. Truly. If you're struggling with excess weight, it's because you're different. You have a different body, which is functioning in a different way and has been on a different life journey to all those people who seem to be able to maintain a healthy weight so effortlessly. It's not your fault.

This book will help you understand the true causes of your weight gain and show you how to reverse it in a responsible way. It will also help you keep that weight off with some easy and effective techniques that are fine-tuned to fit in with your life. By the time you've reached the last page, I hope to have completely changed the way you see the issue of carrying too much fat.

IT'S NOT YOU, IT'S YOUR ENVIRONMENT

Before we go any further, let's take a moment to deal with some of those unhelpful but, sadly, common myths about weight. The Western world has seen soaring levels of obesity since the early eighties. It's easy to jump to the conclusion that people who've been around since then are lazier and greedier than any generation that came before them. This is simply not true and I find it incredible that so many people seem to believe it.

Previous generations weren't trying to be slim. They weren't succeeding where we've failed. They were just going about their daily lives. The same is true for people who live in parts of the world that don't suffer from growing rates of obesity. They're not trying to be slim and managing what we can't. Members of ancient hunter-gatherer tribes, like the ones that we evolved in, weren't trying to be slim. Neither are the members of hunter-gatherer tribes that still exist today. The idea that these people are fundamentally different from us, that they have more motivation and greater willpower, is crazy.

The truth is that evolution works extremely slowly. In other words, humans all over the world have been the same for hundreds of thousands of years. There wasn't a sudden change in the eighties that turned our mindsets fat. What changed was the world around us. No society in the whole of history has been surrounded by as many delicious and tempting calorie-rich foods as we are. On top of that, no previous human society has been expected to do work that requires such little physical activity. Most of us these days spend our working lives behind desks or steering wheels or computer screens and are exposing ourselves to disrupted and irregular sleep routines. We're more tired than ever, more stressed than ever, and more likely to eat outside traditional mealtimes.

All these factors can play a starring role in weight gain. If you put your great-grandparents, or a member of an African tribe that existed a hundred thousand years ago, in a time machine and brought them to our world today, there's every chance that they, too, would develop a problem with excess weight. In other words, it's not us that's changed, it's the world around us.

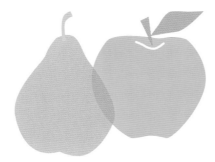

WE ARE ALL DIFFERENT

Ah, you might say, but if it's our environment that's making us fat, and not our laziness or greed, then how come lots of people do manage to stay slim? You can't blame the temptations of the grocery store confectionery aisle or the high-street burger chain or our sedentary lives when we have neighbors, friends, and colleagues who don't seem to struggle like we do.

While it's certainly true that not everyone is carrying excess fat, some of that variation is down to the fact that we're all wired differently. Our genes and past experiences, for example, can help to set the dial on how much we crave unhealthy foods and how our body responds when eating those foods. They can also influence how likely we are to cave at the sight of a chocolate bar at the grocery store checkout. Perhaps you grew up in a family that wasn't able to make healthy choices or you may have a job that makes it really challenging to have a routine around food. Or, maybe your life is full of stress that results in you prioritizing other things, like money and bills, before your health. Perhaps you are a carer for others and feel that you barely have enough time to sleep, let alone think about the quality of the food that you are putting in your mouth. You might live or work in an environment that's more likely to trigger unhealthy eating behaviors. Or, you may have suffered through punishing calorie-restriction diets that have made your problem worse. You could be all of the above.

But don't despair. There is hope. In fact, there's more than just hope. Over the last few years, scientists have made some incredible discoveries, and we're going to take full advantage of them in order to solve your weight problems once and for all.

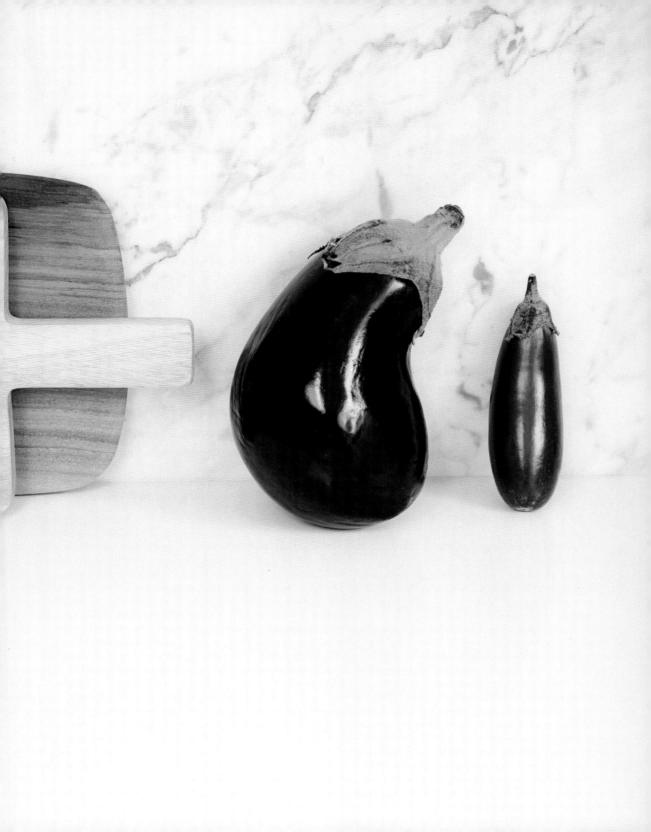

WHY DIETS DON'T WORK

Over the last twenty years of seeing patients, I've witnessed the same thing in my clinic time and time again. People come in full of enthusiasm about some trendy new weight-loss plan, convinced it's the final answer they've been looking for. But when I see them a few months later, they're back to where they started—or worse. It's heartbreaking to witness but it's also, sadly, predictable. Conventional diets usually work only for a short amount of time.

What happens is this: people feel extremely motivated for a while and they follow their diet books to the letter. They succeed in losing weight and they feel amazing. They think they've got it figured out. But here's the secret of the diet-book industry—most of them work okay for three or four weeks and, in that time, everyone talks about the book to everyone else, which drives the sales up. They become bestsellers, which in itself drives even more sales. But a few months later, these latest and greatest books usually quietly disappear from the shelves. By this time, many of their readers will have put all the weight they lost right back on again—and they'll have blamed themselves.

But they shouldn't. They haven't failed; the diet plan they've been following has. Conventional diets generally don't work because they put people on a regime of hunger and willpower that's simply not sustainable. They also fail because they usually tackle only one or two areas of life—what you're eating and how you're moving—rather than treating the whole life and the whole person. Carrying excess weight is usually down to a variety of factors, and they all require care and attention. Finally, they don't really understand what's going on biologically when we're not eating in a healthy way. For the vast majority of people, the core problem has little to do with willpower and exercise and everything to do with the way their bodies are currently working.

IT'S WORTH IT

I sometimes meet patients who've been influenced by the body-positivity movement, which campaigns for the broader acceptance of people, whatever their weight. I completely agree with much of what they're saying. I believe they're right to point out that we live in a fat-phobic society that has all sorts of cruel and inaccurate ideas about larger men and women. However, a small minority of activists go further than this and claim that the science around weight and health outcomes is not accurate, while others encourage people not to do anything about their excess fat.

This can have harmful and unintended consequences. While there's plenty of fascinating debate to be had around these issues, there's no doubt whatsoever among experts that if you are currently carrying excess weight and you become slimmer, you'll be sick less and you'll probably live longer. It's highly likely that your mood and mental health will improve as well.

THE FUEL TANK AND THE FLASHING LIGHT

This is where I'd like to start changing the way you think about your relationship with weight. Think about the food you eat as fuel for your body, just like gas is fuel for your car. If your car detects that it's got an empty fuel tank, it'll flash a light on your dashboard to alert you and tell you to fill up. It's a warning sign. It's a signal that says, "If you don't give me more gas soon, there's going to be a problem. The vehicle will shut down." You can think of your body, and its food system, in just the same way. That flashing warning light is your hunger. It's triggered when your body thinks you're running out of fuel. It tells you, urgently and insistently, that you must fill up with more food, otherwise there's going to be a problem.

But this alarm system can go wrong. Just like in a car, there's a complex mechanism that connects your fuel tank, which includes your stomach and your body's fat stores, to your alarm system, which is your hunger. In the majority of people who are struggling with excess weight, this connection has gone awry. Their flashing light—their hunger—keeps going off when it shouldn't. They're feeling hungry when they don't actually need any more food at all. One reason that many traditional diets fail is because they instruct you to simply ignore this hunger signal, but hunger is one of the most powerful feelings it's possible to experience. It's been a part of us, and has been guiding our behavior and decisions, since the very start of humanity. It's simply not realistic to expect people to just ignore it and go about their day.

Of course, human bodies are a lot more complex than cars. There are further signals that we're not consciously aware of and don't actually physically feel in the way that we feel hunger. These silent signals communicate with different parts of our body and influence what happens to the food that we've consumed—whether it gets burned off as energy or stored as fat.

If you have a problem with excess weight, there's a very high likelihood that you have a malfunction, or a series of malfunctions, in your signalling system. This is why it's not right to blame yourself for your weight gain. When your car breaks down you don't treat it as if it's acted in a sinful way. You understand that your car doesn't have a morale problem that can be put right with a regime of punishing, blaming, and shaming. Just like that car, you're not being weak, lazy, or immoral. You're simply responding appropriately to the signals that your body is giving out. You're eating when you're hungry, stopping when you're not, and storing fat when your body thinks it's appropriate to store fat. You can't control these bodily signals any more than you can control feeling tired after a long day, or hot in the summertime, or in pain when you stub your toe. You're behaving in a perfectly natural way.

This book is packed with solutions that will help you tune these signals correctly and get them back on track so they start working for you, and not against you.

UNDERSTANDING THE WEIGHT POINT

There are lots of things that can damage a person's signalling system. Before we dive into them in more detail, it's important to understand one final, simple concept that we're going to be talking about in the pages to come. Let's go back to our analogy of the car fuel tank. You'll know that different cars have different-sized tanks. A small car might have a tank that can hold about sixteen gallons of fuel, for example, whereas some big four-wheel drives can take more than double that amount. If its signals are to work properly, a car's system has to be programed to know how big its tank is. Why? Because six gallons of fuel in a little Ford Fiesta is plenty, but the same amount in a big Land Rover means it's getting pretty empty. A car can only know to flash its "low fuel" warning signal by first knowing how much fuel it's ideally supposed to carry.

Your body is the same. Your brain has a setting that we're going to call its "weight point." This is the level that it considers to be your ideal weight. If you lose fat, and go below your weight point, your body will make lots of powerful adjustments to its signaling system that trigger you to eat more food and store more of what you eat as fat. If you gain fat, and go too far above your weight point, it'll decide you're carrying too much and make adjustments that trigger you to eat less food and store less of it as fat. If you're carrying excess weight, there's a very good chance that your brain's "ideal weight" is set too high. It's unlikely that you'll be able to lose fat and keep it off until this setting is adjusted downwards.

If you've been on lots of low-calorie diets in the past, your weight point is likely to have changed. This is because, in our evolutionary pasts when our bodies were being designed, weight loss was usually a sign of impending doom. If we were dropping weight, it might have been due to a famine, or perhaps you'd been injured and were finding it difficult to go out and find

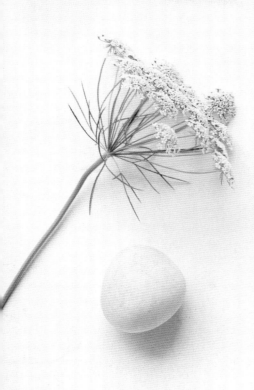

food. So how does your body react? It adjusts your settings in order to protect you. It makes you extra hungry in order to motivate you to get out there and fuel up. It also increases its store-fat settings so you hold on to more fuel in the form of fat. It moves your weight point up, so you carry more fuel around with you every day and are better prepared if things go wrong again in the future.

In other words, it does everything it can to make you fatter. Your system doesn't know you're trying to lose weight on purpose. It's not trying to give you a bad day on your bathroom scales. It's trying to save your life.

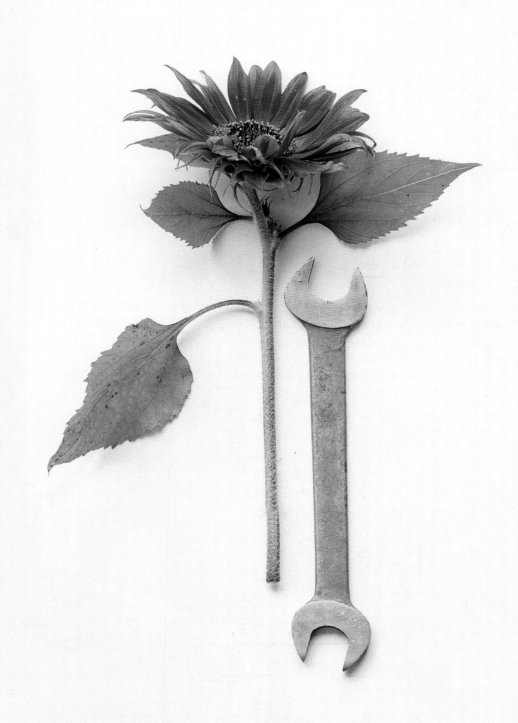

BECOMING YOUR OWN MECHANIC

As you read through this book, I will teach you how to fix your own signals, so your body asks for less food and stores less of what you do eat as fat. I'll also be helping you to dial down your weight point. This will result in you becoming slimmer without suffering from hunger and fatigue. You will lose weight *and* feel great.

Just as every car that goes to the garage with a mechanical issue will have a different history and a different set of problems under the hood, so every patient who walks through my clinic door has their own particular issues. I'm not going to tell you exactly what to do in this book, because I haven't had the opportunity to personally assess you. Instead, I'm going to teach you how to become your own mechanic, so you can design your own made-to-measure weight-loss program.

I have split this book into five separate sections that, I hope, will reframe the way you think about the causes of carrying excess weight. Of course, food is going to feature prominently throughout the book but it is not only *what* you eat that is important—*why* you eat, *when* you eat, *how* you eat, and *where* you eat are critical factors to consider as well.

WHAT WE EAT

Some foods damage your hunger signal, and stop you from feeling full. Some foods increase your cravings, increase your weight point, and over-activate your store-fat signal. Healthy wholefood meals will help reset your body's signals so you eat just enough and feel satisfied.

WHY WE EAT

Lots of people who struggle with their weight eat not because they're hungry for food but because they're hungry for emotional satisfaction. They might be lacking in love for themselves or suffering from too much stress or lack of sleep. This can be tackled by moving in the right way and by learning some simple techniques to make us calm in the day and rest properly at night.

WHEN WE EAT

When we eat can be just as important as what we eat. It's important to understand that the body has daily rhythms, and when we eat out of sync with them, we make it more likely we'll put on excess weight. We should also be careful not to eat too frequently and have set periods in the day where we don't eat in order to help reset our signals.

HOW WE EAT

A lot of us feel constantly busy and seem never to stop rushing around. This results in us not paying attention to our food when we eat. When we do this, we can eat too much and our body doesn't process our food efficiently. Eating mindfully can help decrease the hunger signal and can result in eating less but still feeling satisfied.

WHERE WE EAT

Our environment influences our behavior much more than we think. Simple tweaks to our home and work environments can nudge us into making healthy habits easier to do, while making behaviors we are trying to avoid just that little bit harder.

YOU **CAN** LOSE WEIGHT AND FEEL GREAT

You're worth looking after. You're worth feeling good about. You have a life that's worth protecting and extending. So, please, come with me on this life-changing journey. I'm going to help you lose weight in a responsible way, in a sustainable way and in a way that's going to make you more energetic, will increase your self-esteem, and help you live longer. If it's going to work, this program must be enjoyable, it must not leave you hungry and it must work around your life. This is my recipe for lasting success.

BUILDING YOUR TOOLBOX

As you read through this book, pay attention to the areas which resonate with you the most. Not every section will be relevant to you but it's important you know what they are, so you can decide if they apply to your life situation. Everyone has a different life story, experiences, and relationship with food. Therefore, everyone's individual weight-loss plan will be subtly different as well.

On the page opposite, write down notes and page references for any areas that you think are especially important for you.

At the end of this book, I will put everything together for you and help you design your very own plan that will empower you to lose weight, for good.

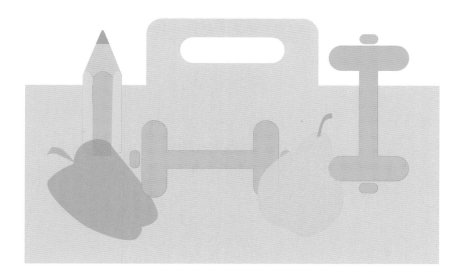

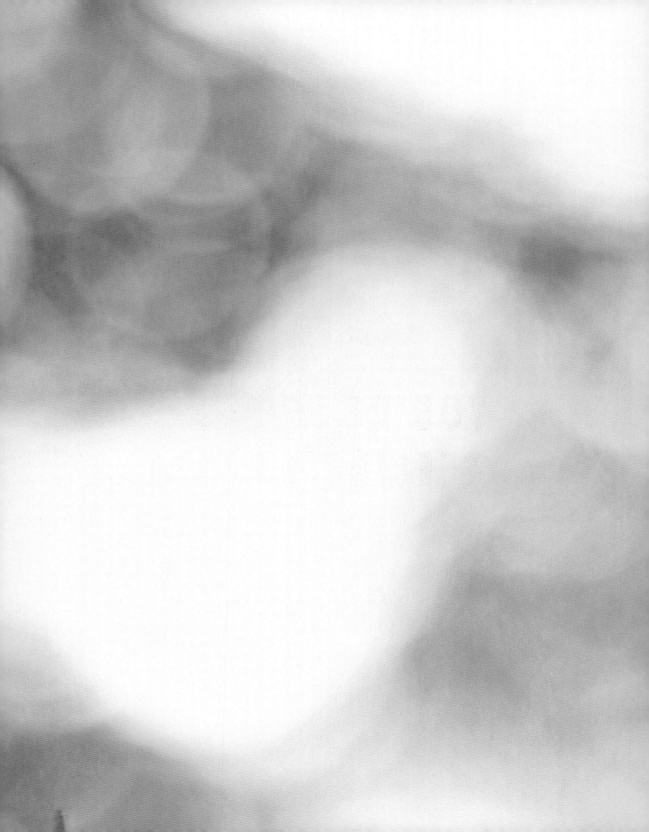

"YOU'RE WORTH LOOKING AFTER. YOU'RE WORTH FEELING GOOD ABOUT."

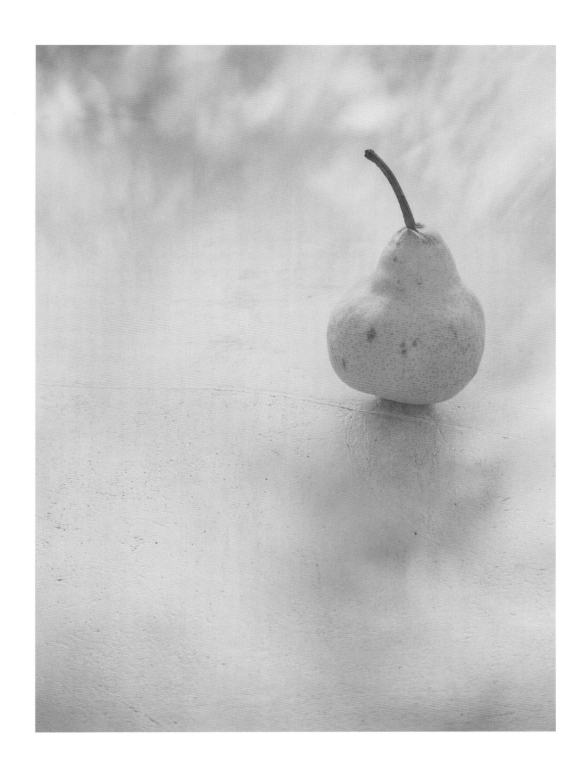

1

WHAT
WE
EAT

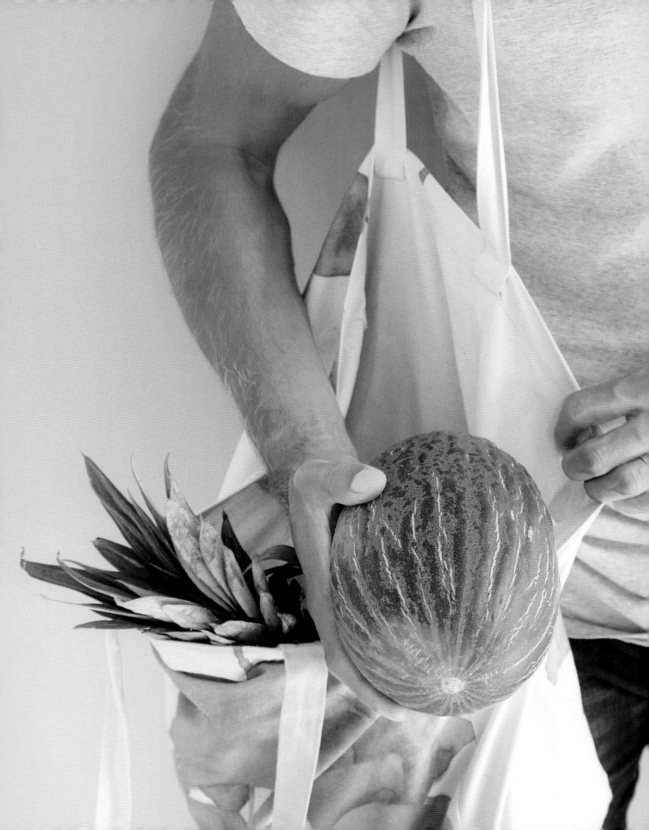

EAT (MORE) REAL FOOD

You're not going to be surprised to hear that food's going to be a major part of your weight-loss journey. That's pretty obvious. I also realize that you don't need me to tell you that eating less sugar and cutting back on pastries is going to be a good idea. You already know that. It's not necessarily a lack of information that's causing you to carry excess weight. We all broadly know what we should and shouldn't eat.

In fact, I'd argue there's too much information out there. Every month there seems to be a new set of rules for healthy eating. One day we're off carbs, the next it's all about paleo or plant-based food. Fats are bad, then fats are good. The problem with all this back and forth is that it can lead us to think, "Well, the experts don't know the answer, so what's the point in trying anything?"

But there are some things we're pretty sure about. And it's going to be hugely valuable to pay attention to them if we're going to succeed in getting healthier and losing weight for good. One of the most important is that *what* we eat is just as important as *how much* we eat—perhaps even more so, because *what* we eat can directly influence *how much* we eat.

Different kinds of food change our body's signals in different ways. As we've already discovered, it's the signals our body gives out that drive our food choices and behavior. Mastering weight loss means controlling these powerful hunger and store-fat signals so we can lose fat without having to rely on willpower alone.

In almost twenty years of seeing patients, I've learned that one of the most powerful pieces of health advice I can give anyone is this: **eat (more) real food**.

What I mean by "real food" is food that's minimally processed, close to its natural state and instantly recognizable—fish that looks like fish, meat that looks like meat, vegetables that look like vegetables, etc.

It's often the biggest game-changer and leads to people feeling better in every way: mind, body, and heart.

This one simple habit has three almost magical benefits:

1
You'll feel less hungry.

2
Your body will automatically manage your weight for you.

3
You'll be less tempted to eat what I call "blissy foods."

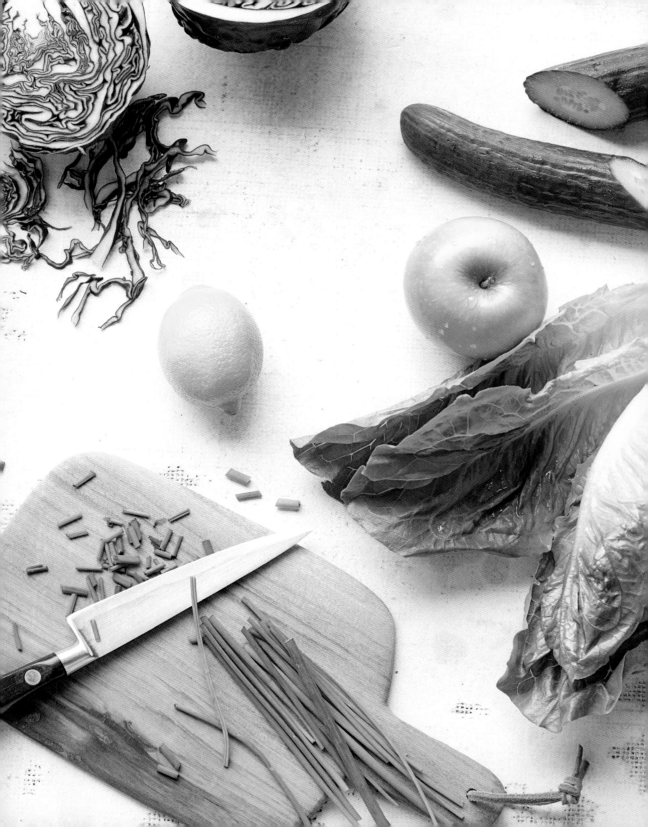

BLISSY FOODS

So, what are "blissy foods?" These are products that are about as far away as possible from the real foods I'd like you to eat. They're often created by scientists who know that certain kinds of foods have powerful effects on our hunger signals. This is how they make their products so devilishly successful. Anyone determined to eat healthily is pitting themselves against teams of incredibly smart people who've spent decades designing foods that are utterly irresistible to the human brain. These chocolate bars, chips, sweets, and salty, fatty meals have been engineered to hammer at your hunger signals. Food manufacturers know that when you open that bag of chips it will be extremely hard to stop eating them, and that one chunk of chocolate can so easily lead to eating the whole bar. They know this happens because these foods have been deliberately built that way.

This is how it works. Our brains are wired to uniquely respond to a few specific properties in food, including certain kinds of carbs, starch, sugar, protein, fat, salt, and the savory "umami" flavor which is found in foods like cooked meats, broths, and seaweed. When our food contains these flavors in certain combinations, the brain releases a chemical called dopamine. This dopamine has a powerful effect on our behavior and impacts the food choices that we make. In fact, once we've eaten these foods and experienced the "bliss" they provide, our brains will even release dopamine in *anticipation* of eating these foods again. The job of dopamine is to teach us how to do important things like satisfy our hunger. Some call it the learning molecule. Dopamine helps create intense feelings of reward, and this motivates us to repeat the same behavior—eating those blissy foods—over and over again.

The foods that cause the highest spike in dopamine levels tend to be ones that are exceptionally full of calories. The more often we satisfy our cravings with these blissy foods, the more we'll experience that dopamine hit and the more powerfully the lesson will be reinforced: when we're hungry, we should seek out blissy foods. Eventually, the programming in our brain becomes so powerful it's practically automatic. The mere smell or even the sight of the familiar packaging of these foods can trigger our behavior, as our brain takes over, running the unconscious sequence of behaviors that it's learned to use to satisfy itself. Even being in the location where you last had that food will trigger the release of dopamine.

It may feel like your brain's working against you, but it's actually trying to help. It's wired to seek out as much high-calorie food as possible so it can keep you alive, and it tries to predict the best course of action based upon your past behavior. If you satisfy hunger at the cookie jar, then that's where it'll send you when you're hungry. This is why it's so hard to resist that packet of chocolate-chip cookies or smoky-bacon chips that are in your cupboard. As soon as you feel tired or peckish, your brain will begin the program of taking you there and opening the packet. Your brain remembers your past experience and so dopamine spikes even before you start eating it. If merely reading the words "chocolate-chip cookies" or "smoky-bacon chips" is making you feel edgy, tempted, and hungry, it's happening to you right now.

In the junk-food business there's even a technical term—"bliss point"—that describes the perfect combination of tastes and textures that makes a product irresistible. These technicians have discovered that the dopamine in our brain surges a lot more when these special properties, like sweet and salty, are put together in a combination. Fifty years ago, who had ever heard of putting salt on caramel? Now, you see combinations like this everywhere—in cakes, in syrups, in cookies, in toppings for your ice cream. As soon as these two flavors were put together, it spread like wildfire. The invention of salted caramel was another huge success in the efforts of food manufacturers to hijack the brain signals of the ordinary person on the street.

The signals that blissy foods like salted caramel and smoky-bacon chips—or, my own favorite, shortbread—trigger are tremendously powerful because they're ancient. They've been wired into our brains over tens of thousands of years. For the vast majority of the time humans have been on Earth, food has been extremely hard to come by. Up until recently, for some of our ancestors, it was a genuinely difficult feat to survive long, freezing winters, and it was normal for a proportion of the elderly and the very young to sometimes not make it through the cold season. This is why the brain is wired to crave food when it seems available and abundant—and especially food that's packed full of calories. It's trying to keep us alive. The problem is, this kind of calorie-dense food is both more available, and cheaper to buy, than it's ever been before in human history.

We're surrounded by blissy foods that have been designed to trigger our cravings and I know from my patients just how effective they can be. Billie, 37, worked hard in human resources and struggled for years, jumping from diet to diet. She'd drive home from the office each night between 6.30 p.m. and 7 p.m., her best route taking her past a particular roundabout where the smell of junk food was overwhelming. At least three times a week, without quite knowing how, she'd find herself in line for the drive-thru. She "knew" eating fries and chicken tenders wouldn't help her weight, and felt determined to eat more healthily, but her brain and body had other ideas. She'd beat herself up afterwards, calling herself "pathetic" and "weak," and swear that the next day she'd have the strength to drive on by. When she came in to see me full of shame and regret, I had to tell her that it wasn't her fault. She was responding, perfectly naturally, to the release of dopamine in her brain. It was going to be near impossible to fight. Because, believe it or not, it's the same chemical that's released in the brains of gamblers and drug addicts.

I explained that her best solution might be to take a different route home, even if it did take 20 minutes longer. That's exactly what she did, and that one simple change led to Billie eating more home-cooked meals and, ultimately, losing her excess weight.

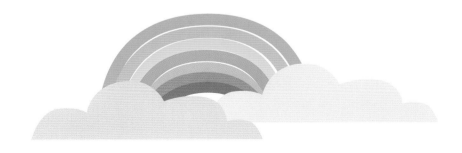

ADDICTED TO BLISS?

Does this mean we crave junk food in the same way we might crave alcohol, nicotine, or even cocaine? Can blissy food be truly addictive? I'm the first to acknowledge that the concept of food addiction is controversial, but we do know enough about these blissy foods to say that they're extremely hard to resist and that millions of people struggle to do so every day. We also know that the brain systems that are involved with craving, enjoying, and repeating the experience of eating junk food are the same as the systems that are involved with craving, enjoying, and repeating the experience of taking drugs.

To me, whether or not our behavior around blissy foods can technically be called an addiction is of little importance. We should let the academics fight among themselves about the exact use of the term. What we can say with absolute certainty is that these foods have an addictive-like quality and they trigger addiction-like behaviors.

Blissy foods have become such an ordinary part of our lives that we're now told that even so-called healthy foods should have their irresistible qualities. There's a huge and growing business in books that want to teach us how to make low-calorie food as delicious as possible. While I understand the rationale behind this, I do have reservations. Not everything has to be overwhelmingly delicious. In fact, we're making things much harder for ourselves if it is.

When we were evolving in our hunter-gatherer tribes, the food we ate was often bland and repetitive, and this would have helped keep our signals working properly. Of course, I'm not saying you have to eat plain porridge for every meal, just as I'm not saying you can never eat ice cream again. But neither do I think you should be striving to make all your daily, ordinary meals mind-blowingly tasty. The constant entertainment of the taste buds that we're sometimes pressured to experience has become part of the problem. There's no shame in eating mostly simple, straightforward meals that taste good enough. Saving your blissy foods for special occasions will be a huge help in fixing your damaged signals.

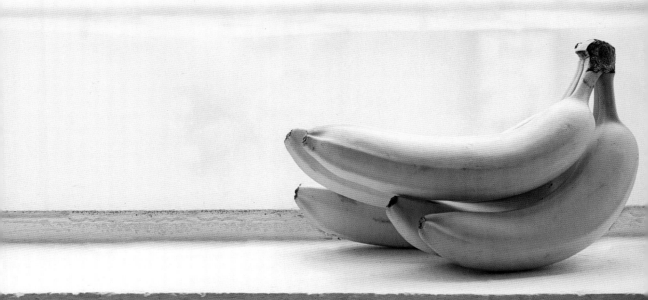

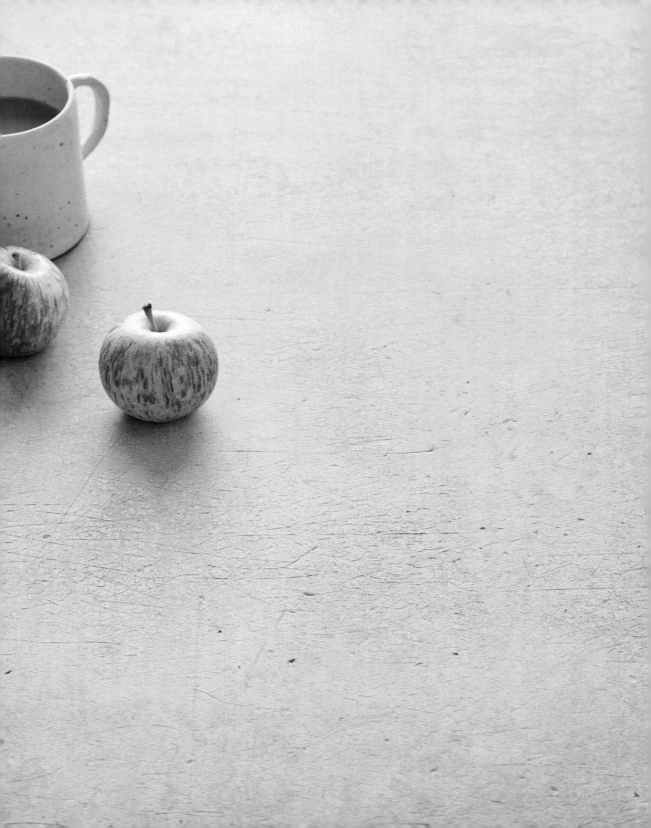

THE BUFFET EFFECT

We all know that feeling when we're completely full and we're sure we can't stuff another morsel in our mouths—until dessert comes out. Suddenly we have an extra compartment ready. What's going on? The scientific term for this is "sensory-specific satiety." This basically means that we can feel full for one type of flavor—something savory, spicy, or sweet—and yet still have an appetite for another. Some people also call this the "buffet effect." Buffets are notorious for encouraging us to overeat. Because there's such a huge array of different flavors laid out in front of us, it ramps up the likelihood we'll keep going back for more.

I noticed this playing out at the start of the 2020 pandemic. My family were having three home-cooked meals per day and, of course, were unable to visit cafés or restaurants, because they were closed. After a while, the food started to become a bit monotonous and, as a result, I just naturally ended up eating less. We would have a few core meals we'd repeat in sequence over and over again. We enjoyed them, for sure. But because we couldn't spice things up regularly with takeout, we naturally ended up eating less.

People who live in some of the healthiest regions of the world, where they tend to be able to keep excess weight off effortlessly, experience something similar. They have a core group of recipes they use over and over again. They don't have the option to constantly seek out new flavors or face pressure to do so from social media and trendy recipe books.

What would you choose as your core healthy wholefood ingredients that you can design all your food around? Why not challenge yourself to spend three weeks, or longer, cooking only from those, while avoiding takeout, and pay attention to how this makes you feel?

(If a need for sweetness after each meal is a habit that keeps tripping you up, get into the habit of eating a piece of fruit.)

THE WONKY HUNGER SIGNAL

If you want to achieve weight loss that actually lasts, you have to work *with* your body's signals, not *against* them. You have to control hunger. If you've been making a habit of eating blissy foods, there's a very good chance that your hunger signal isn't working properly.

One of the ways it can go wrong is by failing to signal when we're full. Over time, this feeling of satisfaction is largely the job of a chemical called leptin that's released into the blood by our fat cells. Leptin says to our bodies, "You are already carrying enough fat. You don't need to take extra fuel on board." But many of us now find it hard to pick these critical leptin signals up. Just as listening to loud music over a long period can make our ears deaf to sounds, eating lots of processed food can make our brains deaf to leptin. We don't feel full when our body actually *is* full. This phenomenon is extremely common these days and is called "leptin resistance." It's one of the main causes of excess weight gain. Leptin is the most important hormone in your body when it comes to how much fat you store. Period. Therefore, having this hormone work well, in a way that helps you rather than harms you, is crucial.

So, how does eating large quantities of blissy, highly processed foods make us deaf to leptin? Firstly, these foods usually contain a combination of highly refined carbohydrates and oils that can cause the body to flip itself into a special survival mode called inflammation. When we're in this mode, the body struggles to hear the leptin signal because it's focusing on other priorities. In addition, the refined oils that these foods contain interfere with the body's crucial ability to switch any inflammation off.

Secondly, when we eat highly processed foods that contain lots of refined carbohydrates, our systems release unusually large amounts of a hormone called insulin, compared to when we are eating minimally processed wholefoods. Insulin helps us to direct where the energy in our food goes and where it gets stored in the body. But when we have large and persistent increases in insulin from regularly eating and snacking on blissy processed foods, it travels to the brain and interferes with the signal from leptin. The result? We don't feel full when we should. Baked goods—such as croissants, pastries, cakes, cookies, and most supermarket breads*—are particularly problematic in this regard. They tend to be exceptionally high in calories, cause large spikes in insulin, and play havoc with blood sugar levels. They often leave you feeling tired, moody, and hungry and, in my experience, should be minimized as much as possible if you are trying to lose weight.

The great news is we can repair this leptin resistance fairly easily, by eating food the body recognizes as food. This is why the quality of our meals, and the ingredients we put in them, is of such huge importance. We can only stop eating too much when we feel full at the right times. It's also important that we don't over-complicate our diets with long lists of "good" and "bad" foods. Perhaps the most straightforward way of thinking about it is that we want to eat one-ingredient foods and meals that are made out of a small number of single ingredients.

* If you do wish to eat bread, try to choose ones that are made with proper wholegrains, have ingredients that you can easily recognize, and are made in a traditional style. Good options tend to be the dark German-style breads that are full of seeds and often come in squares.

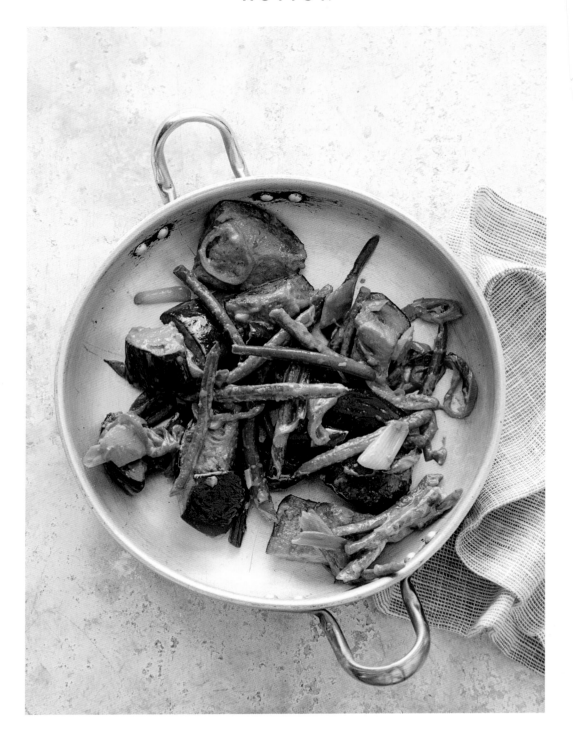

FOCUS ON ONE-INGREDIENT FOODS

Try to eat more foods that don't come with ingredient labels

I'd like you to eat more real food by focusing on one-ingredient foods. These are foods that don't tend to come with ingredient labels. Examples include carrots, apples, potatoes, avocados, fish, eggs, and beans. Have you ever noticed that we don't form habits and cravings for these types of foods? Try your best to ensure that the majority of your diet is made up of foods like these—either eaten by themselves or combined together in simple wholefood meals.

These simple, real foods don't naturally come in blissy combinations of fat-salt-sweet. They're not designed in a laboratory to stimulate the dopamine-releasing regions of the brain. Nor do they drive up levels of inflammation in the body and play havoc with the body's natural hunger and fullness signals. In effect, they work with your body and not against it.

6 TIPS TO HELP YOU EAT MORE ONE-INGREDIENT FOODS

1

Shop on the outermost aisles of the supermarket.
Most one-ingredient foods tend to live here. This is a tip I have borrowed from the brilliant food writer Michael Pollan.

2

Keep frozen vegetables in the house at all times.
They are easy to steam, cheap to buy, and can be super tasty, especially with the simple addition of herbs and spices.

3

Keep chopped garlic and onions in the fridge or freezer to speed up cooking and preparation time.

4

Use herbs and spices freely.
They are a simple and healthy way to add more flavor to real-food meals.

5

Stock up on one-ingredient store cupboard essentials such as canned tomatoes, canned fish, coconut milk, lentils, beans, brown rice, nuts, etc.—so you always have something at hand when hungry or ready to cook.

6

Batch cook on the weekends (or another convenient time) so you always have real-food options for later in the week when you may have less time.

INGREDIENT LABELS: A SIMPLE RULE

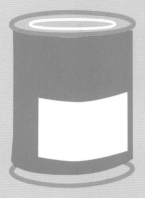

For anyone keen to increase the general quality of their food intake, it's a great idea to get into the habit of looking at the ingredient labels on everything you buy. One-ingredient foods, such as fresh fish, meat, and vegetables don't tend to have labels because what you're seeing is what you're getting. But packaged food often has long lists of ingredients, some of which will be hard to recognize or even pronounce. A good rule of thumb is to try and avoid foods that contain these gobbledegook ingredients, or that have more than five ingredients in total. Things are not quite this simple in reality—sometimes those gobbledegook words are just technical language for ingredients that are okay. But living by this simple rule will dramatically reduce your consumption of the kinds of foods that have the potential to play havoc with your body's hunger and fullness signals.

Of course, it's completely fine for us to create meals at home that contain more than five wholefood ingredients!

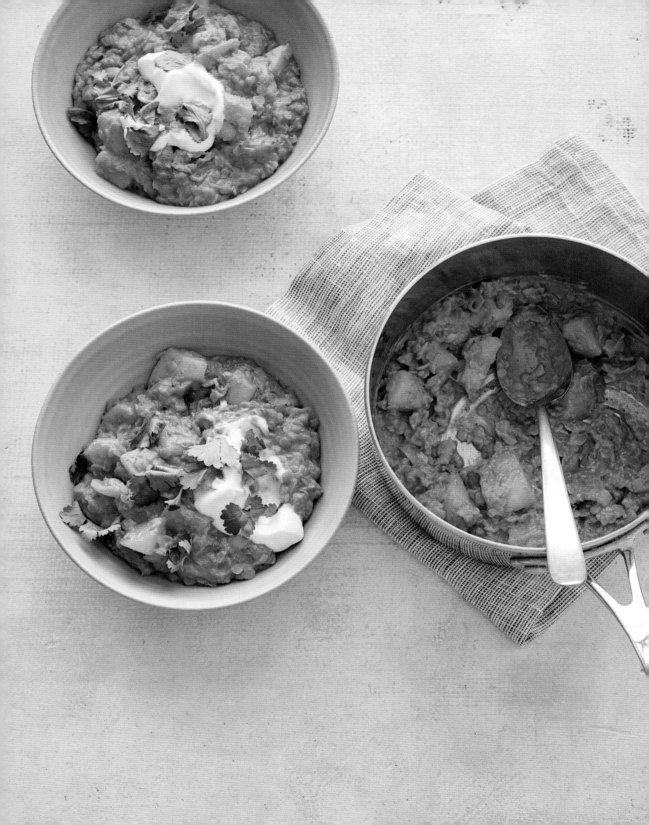

FORGET THE PERFECT DIET

There's no one perfect diet. Everybody is different. We all have different bodies and brains that give out different signals at different strengths and in different circumstances. You might have friends who've lost weight on the paleo diet; you might have friends who've lost weight going vegan, or on a low-fat or no-carb regime. Each of these friends might swear by their method, convinced it's the only one that really works. But what does all this really tell us? It tells us that different things work for different people.

There are some common principles that seem to apply to all health-promoting diets. One of them is that they are mostly made up of minimally processed foods—in other words, foods that, when they're on your plate, are as close to their natural state as possible. Think of a roast dinner—a leg of lamb, some roasted potatoes, and some veggies. Or, if you choose to be vegan, think about a plate of black beans, sweet potato, and broccoli, or a bowl of dahl and rice. That is real food, the sort of food we've been eating for millennia. Contrast that with a ready meal you shove in your microwave that contains twenty ingredients you don't recognize and which sends your body's signals haywire.

In one scientific study, people spent two weeks with unlimited access to highly processed "blissy" foods and another two weeks with unlimited access to freshly cooked food made from whole ingredients. Both of the diets had the same amount of calories, fiber, sugar, and fat. Both were rated as equally enjoyable and tasty. But the people in the study ate up to 500 calories extra of the "blissy" processed-food diet, every single day. It messed up their hunger and fullness signals, so they didn't know when to stop. That's the equivalent of 15,000 calories a month, and an astonishing 180,000 calories a year.

What this shows us is that wholefoods work with your signals properly, while blissy foods mess them up. What's more, they help to lower your body's weight point (see box opposite), which is the size your brain thinks you ought to be and will fight to keep you at. If you have a low weight point, it means your body will do the hard work of taking your excess fat off for you, and you will find it effortless.

One of the best strategies to lower your weight point is to eat a real-food diet consistently. If you are to sustain this way of eating over the long term, it's important that your food choices don't end up being too difficult for you to stick to. Be realistic and try to find a way of eating minimally processed food that you enjoy, that you find simple to prepare, and that makes you feel full. When you manage this (and you absolutely will!), you will find weight loss effortless and sustainable.

THE WEIGHT POINT

You've probably heard of the reality show *The Biggest Loser*, which pits dieters against each other to see who can drop the most weight. When researchers studied the contestants, they found this process actually worked against most of them in the long term. One *Biggest Loser* star automatically burned about 2,500 calories a day when he arrived on the show. But two years later, after all that grueling weight loss, his body was burning just 1,400 calories a day. In other words, his weight point hadn't budged. His brain still thought he was supposed to be incredibly heavy and so slowed down his entire system to make it more efficient and to burn fewer calories.

I've seen this happen time and again in my clinic. One patient, Graham, managed to lose weight by forcibly reducing his calories for about six months. Then he hit a plateau. He loved the way he looked in the mirror but didn't really like himself—and neither did his wife. He felt constantly tired, sluggish, and irritable, and this mood change was affecting his marriage and his ability to do his job.

I explained to Graham what was happening. His body thought that he wasn't getting enough fuel on board. To compensate for this, it had to turn the dial down on Graham's life. That's why he felt weary and moody and hangry and cold and struggled to get out of bed each morning. Everything was working against him in order to try to have him put the fat back on and get him back to his weight point—and he felt absolutely terrible. What he needed to learn was that harsh dieting isn't the answer. Eating the right foods, in sensible amounts, is.

LOW CARB, PLANT-BASED, OR PALEO?

My job as a doctor is to help each and every single one of my patients around their individual desires, ethical preferences, and beliefs. In almost twenty years of clinical practice, I have seen tens of thousands of patients and, truthfully, have seen patients thrive on a variety of different diets. That is why I am diet agnostic and have no preference as to the eating style you adopt.

My main focus when it comes to food is to aim, as much as possible, for minimally processed food. For the vast majority of my patients, this is all they need to do. As well as helping you to control your weight without constantly fighting hunger, diets rich in minimally processed foods have other rather pleasant side effects—they help reduce inflammation in the body, which can help improve a variety of other symptoms such as joint pain, energy levels, mood problems, and sleep quality.

FOOD CHOICES AND THE ENVIRONMENT

When it comes to our food choices, there is also an important discussion to be had around the impact they have on the environment. A detailed discussion on this topic is beyond the scope of this book, as there are many complexities to consider. However, one thing that pretty much all experts agree on is the detrimental impact of factory farming—both from an animal-cruelty perspective and an environmental one—so I would urge you to avoid buying foods that support this practice.

LOW CARB

Some of my patients have done amazingly well on what are commonly known as "low-carb" diets. Those who thrive tend to find that this way of eating helps them feel effortlessly full. They don't feel the urge to snack and consequently find it easier to eat less. Of course, as with any diet, it is possible to do "low carb" badly and fill up with low-carb junk foods. If you're keen to give it a go, I'd recommend you focus on real foods such as non-starchy fiber-rich vegetables, high-quality protein such as fatty fish, responsibly sourced meat, and food like tofu, if you are vegan.

PLANT-BASED

I've also seen people achieve amazing results with a plant-based whole-food diet that is rich in high-quality complex carbohydrates. One particular study on this way of eating, the BROAD study, has shown some of the best weight-loss results I have seen both in the short term and in the long term. Remarkably, in this study, people were allowed to eat as much as they wanted and still managed significant weight loss. This is one of the beautiful side effects of diets based on minimally processed food: you can eat until you're full, and that makes them sustainable.

PALEO

One of my patients followed a paleo-type diet and also got phenomenal results. The idea behind this way of eating is that we go back to eating what our ancestors ate for the bulk of our evolution. For all the criticism of it, I think the basic premise of paleo is robust, but I will say it is probably overly restrictive for many. This patient loved this way of eating and thrived on the way it made him feel. He never felt he had to "restrict" how much he ate, nor did he ever feel he was fighting hunger.

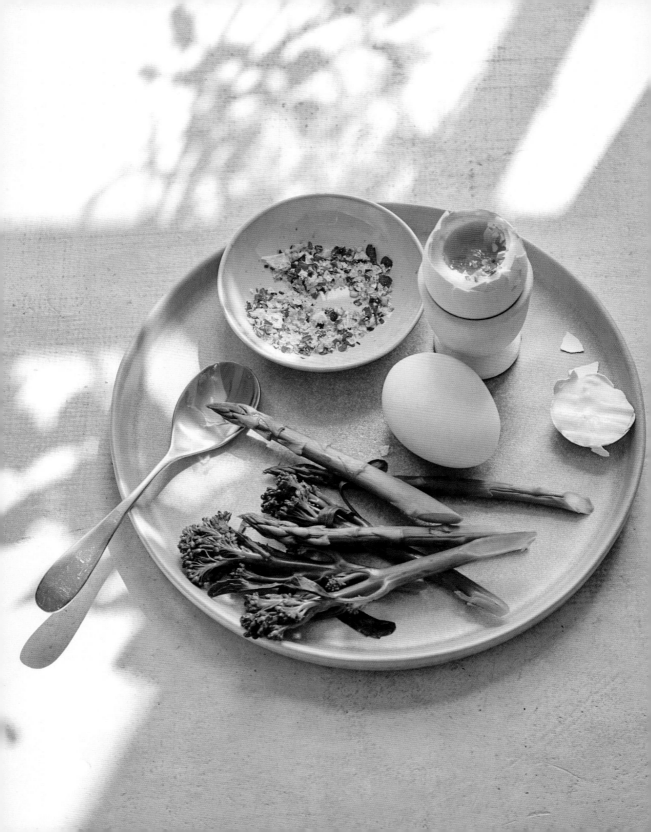

FIXING YOUR FIRST MEAL

Picture this common scenario. You wake up and eat a bowl of cereal: some healthy-looking granola, say, with a dollop of low-fat yogurt. Your stomach stretches, your hunger signal switches off, and you feel satisfied and full. But two hours later, you're going about your day, and you're suddenly starving again. You go to the kitchen to make a cup of tea and, while the kettle's boiling, can't resist the temptation of a few cookies or perhaps a large banana. You're full again. But at twelve thirty, just before lunch, you're not only ravenous, you're also feeling shaky. You pop down the main street and, having planned on getting a healthy salad, you somehow find yourself with a meal deal: sandwich, chips, and a snack bar. By three o'clock you're tired, irritable—and hungry again. A can of cola and another banana will sort you out . . . at least until five thirty, when you're shaky and starving yet again.

This was the daily experience of a patient of mine called Alan. He was vegetarian and generally considered himself pretty healthy, so he couldn't understand why he was finding it so hard to shift the spare tire around his waist. I had to tell him his problem was pretty simple. He was not actually in control of his diet; his blood sugar was. It was taking him on a crazy daily rollercoaster of short, filling highs and deep, shocking crashes. There was little chance of him losing his excess weight until he stepped off that wild sugar ride and reclaimed control over what he put into his mouth.

I explained to Alan that it all began with his granola breakfast. That stuff was full of sugar. As soon as he ate it, the sugar was absorbed into his blood and began racing around his system. In order to bring his blood sugar down, his body released a chemical called insulin, which would start moving that sugar out of the blood and into other parts of his body, as well as stopping the breakdown of any fat. But when the body releases lots of insulin to deal with a big sugar dump, it can often result in blood sugar tumbling far too quickly. This left Alan feeling starving, weak, and shaky. Stress hormones began to flood his body. Because his system was now craving sugar, he headed to the cupboard, or the refrigerator, to seek out something sugary—which started the whole process again.

To get him off the blood-sugar rollercoaster, I suggested something radical. I told Alan to have his dinner for breakfast. He chose to have a large plate of goat's cheese with roasted zucchini, peppers, and sweet potatoes before work every morning. To say he found this life-changing is an understatement. On the first day he got to 2 p.m. before realizing he'd missed lunch. This had never happened before. He didn't feel hungry. He didn't feel snappy or shaky. His concentration levels were high. He used to think he performed well at work, but after a few weeks of his new dinner-breakfast he realized his work had been seriously sub-par. His cognition was now in a different league—and he finally lost that spare tire.

Changing his breakfast changed Alan's whole life. That granola used to sabotage his entire day. All his subsequent food decisions were a domino effect of his breakfast, and it impacted his mood and his performance at work. And the weight started to fall off. Effortlessly. He was also thrilled by how his taste buds automatically changed. Within weeks, a can of cola that used to "hit the spot" now seemed sickly-sweet. He lost fat from his body without really trying and without fighting hunger!

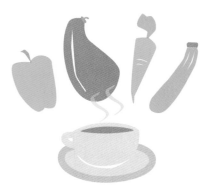

DINNER FOR BREAKFAST

Try having your "dinner foods" for breakfast

I'd like you to experiment with eating foods at breakfast that you might typically only have for dinner. Many of us have fixed ideas about breakfast and only consider options such as sugary cereals, toast, or croissants. This is a mistake because the first meal you eat can set the tone for the rest of the day. It can impact your mood, your concentration, your hunger, and have a powerful influence on your subsequent choices. Why not try some of the following options or come up with your own suggestions instead:

- Goat's cheese with roasted zucchini, peppers, and sweet potatoes

- Leftover roast dinner

- Eggs, broccoli, and potatoes

- Salmon and vegetables

- Dahl and rice

This might take a bit of extra planning at the very start of the day, but the domino effects can be truly life-changing. This doesn't actually need to take as long as you might think. Many of my patients have started to cook extra amounts at dinner the night before, so they can simply pop the leftovers in the fridge overnight and reheat in the morning.

Please remember that there's no one solution that's perfect for everyone, and some prefer not to eat breakfast at all and still feel fine (more on this on page 170). But let's just take a moment to remember what "breakfast" actually means. It's basically when you break your fast. So, yes, that could mean you eat it at 7 a.m. But if you skip traditional "breakfast" and eat your first meal at lunchtime, this is also when you break your fast!

POWER UP WITH PROTEIN

Prioritize protein with every meal

While my overall rule is to simply eat real food, there is one kind of food that deserves special attention when it comes to losing fat, and that's protein. There are three main reasons I recommend eating more protein:

Firstly, it is well established that protein is extremely satiating, which means that it will help you feel full sooner than fat or carbs. Secondly, digesting protein utilizes more energy than other foods, which is really helpful when trying to lose weight. And, thirdly, protein helps maintain muscle mass, and the more of that you have, the more likely it is that your weight point will move down and stay there.

One of the reasons scientists think we eat ultra-processed foods in such high quantities is that we'll keep on eating until we've had enough protein. Blissy foods tend to be low in protein, so it takes a lot of them to satisfy us. Some of my patients who've struggled to lose weight even when consuming real-food diets have achieved remarkable results simply by increasing their protein intake.

As important as protein is, I would urge a note of caution on some high-protein foods such as nuts and nut butters. Although they contain decent amounts of protein, they also come packed with a lot of calories as well, which means you can end up consuming a lot of excess energy alongside the protein if you eat too many of them. Incorporating these foods in your diet can absolutely be helpful when trying to lose weight, but do be careful not to go overboard with them as I have seen many people do when transitioning to real-food diets.

So, how much protein should you consume? This is highly individual, and I would encourage you to use your hand as an initial guide. For men, aim for two palm-sized portions of protein with each meal; and for women, aim for one. Of course, this is only a rough guide. As with everything in this book, you will need to experiment a little to find the right amount for you.

I'd recommend the following sources of protein, depending on your tastes and preferences:

- Lean meats

- Eggs

- Fish

- Greek yogurt

- Pulses, such as lentils and beans

- Beans

- Seeds and unsalted nuts

- Tofu

- Fermented soy products, like seitan and tempeh

- Meat substitutes

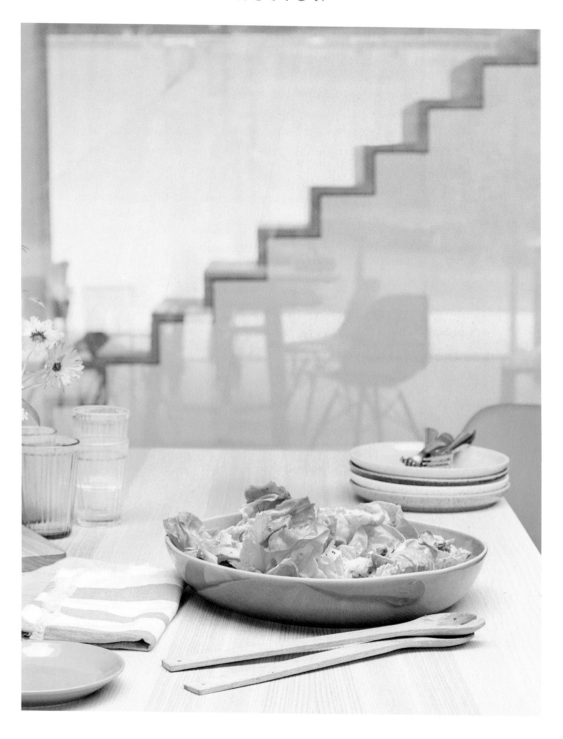

GREENS GO FIRST

Eat salad and vegetables first

This is one of my all-time favorite food tips. I've been using it with my patients (and my kids!) for years. Eating salads and vegetables before tucking into more calorific foods is such an easy hack and can nudge us into eating more of what's beneficial and less of what's not. Salads are full of volume and fiber so they help to fill you up without you taking on a large amount of calories. A salad is also hard to eat quickly. This naturally results in us eating more slowly, which helps us to tune into our hunger and fullness signals (see page 201). Research shows that starting a meal with a leafy green salad can lead to us consuming fewer calories overall. And they don't need to be boring. Salads can be fun and colorful and they have many health benefits on top of being great for weight loss.

The same principle applies to vegetables. When I give my seven-year-old daughter a plate of pan-fried salmon, sweet-potato wedges, and kale, she'll usually eat up the wedges and salmon first and tell me she has no more room for the kale. But when I give her a plate of kale first and tell her she can only have the rest when she's finished it, she miraculously manages to eat up every last bit of kale and then needs less of the other food afterwards.

NB. I do appreciate that some people with digestive ailments, like IBS, often cannot tolerate certain vegetables. My top tip would be to experiment and, initially, stick only to those vegetables you can tolerate. It's important to understand that unmanaged stress is a common trigger for IBS symptoms; the tips in "How We Eat" on pages 185–210 may prove helpful. If you are really struggling, I would recommend seeing a health-care professional for personalized advice.

QUENCH YOUR HUNGER

Drink a glass of water thirty minutes before each meal

Sometimes we can get our signals confused and feel hungry when we're actually thirsty. I've seen countless patients for whom simply drinking a large glass of water thirty minutes before each meal has resulted in them feeling less hungry and eating less. Like so much of the advice in this book, this has benefits that go far beyond weight loss. Many of us don't drink enough water period. Increasing your intake can give you more energy, better concentration, and improved overall health. In addition, drinking lots of water means you'll have to get up more to pee, which increases how much you move around in a day!

While everyone is different, I'd recommend you aim to have at least 48 ounces of water per day. One of the most effective ways to do this is to keep a 24-ounce water bottle with you. Fill it up in the morning and make sure you have drunk the whole bottle by lunchtime. Then, simply refill it and make sure it is empty by dinnertime. Large quantities of water after 6 p.m. can disrupt sleep, so are best avoided.

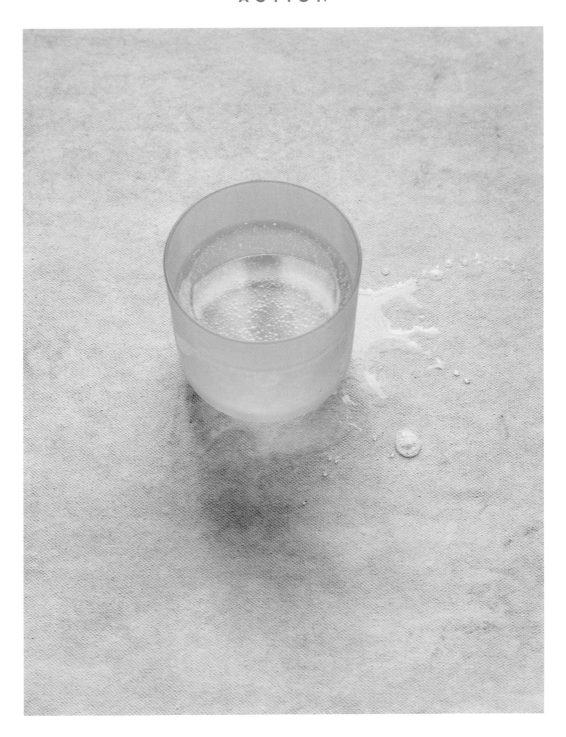

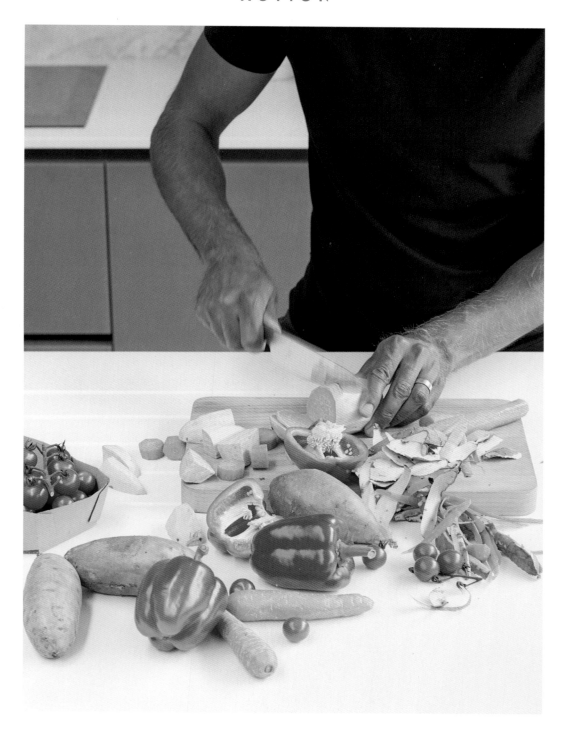

LEARN TO COOK

Learn to cook five wholefood meals that you enjoy

It's an odd world we live in when we spend more time watching cookery shows than actually cooking. I've got nothing against these programs, and have even appeared in one or two of them myself. However, I do think they say something fascinating about our relationship with food. We're using it for purposes it has not been designed for. Food has become entertainment and a status symbol. It's something we compete over, whether we're a contestant on *The Great British Bake Off* or snapping a shot of our breakfast to post on social media.

The danger is that we'll feel pressured to ensure every meal we eat is as pretty as a picture and delicious enough for a TV judge. We lose our grip on the simple fact that food is nourishment as well as fuel for our bodies and minds. It doesn't have to be eye-poppingly tasty every time we sit down to eat and, if it is, we're likely to mess up our signals and eat much more than is healthy. If we're going to have sustainable weight loss, we're going to have to get used to eating food that's tasty enough and made from wholefoods. This means doing a bit of simple cooking from scratch.

If you don't know how to cook, I would strongly urge you to learn. It really does not need to be complicated. There are some fabulous recipe books and YouTube videos out there that will teach you the basics—invest some time in finding resources that you like and challenge yourself to learn five simple and quick wholefood-based meals that you enjoy.

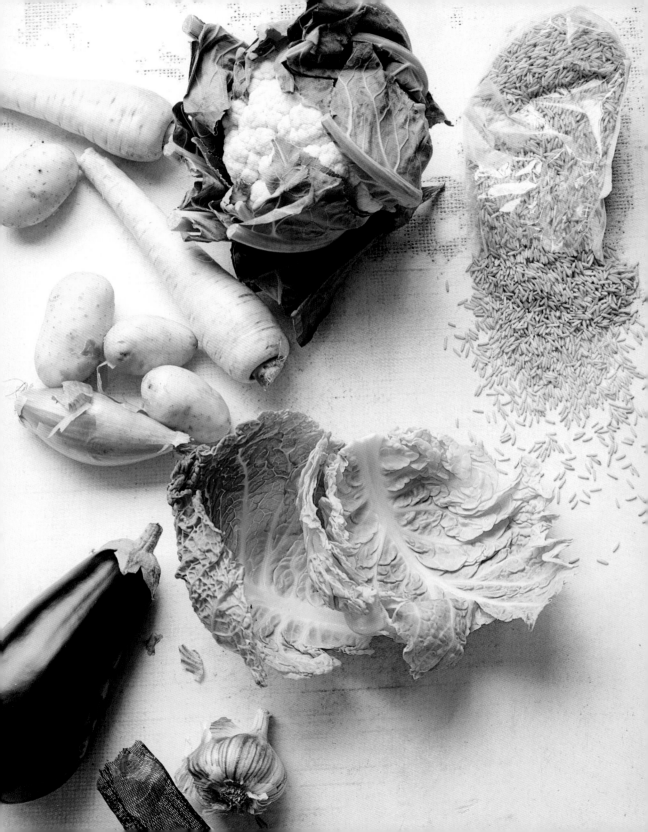

WHOLEFOODS TO BASE YOUR MEALS AND SNACKS AROUND

Whatever dietary preference you have, basing your meals around wholefoods will help you improve your health and lose weight. Below is a list of wholefoods that I would recommend you create your meals from. You don't need to be completely rigid and inflexible about this. Use this as a guide only and, please remember, this is not an exhaustive list.

- **Vegetables**—fresh and frozen
- **Fruit**—fresh and canned (if canned, watch out for added sugar)
- **Wholegrains** such as buckwheat, brown rice, quinoa, and spelt
- **Lean Meat**
- **Fish**—canned or fresh
- **Eggs**
- **Nuts and seeds**
- **Pulses** such as lentils, peas, and beans. Examples include black beans, pinto beans, butter beans, chickpeas, kidney beans, and black-eyed beans
- **Herbs and spices** such as ginger, turmeric, and cumin can be used freely to enhance flavor

As you can see from the list above, you do not always need to eat fresh wholefoods. For example, frozen vegetables can be very helpful, as they can live in your freezer, chopped and ready to throw into a variety of recipes. In addition, they often have more nutrients within them than fresh vegetables, as they are frozen soon after picking. Buying ready-made wholefoods such as hummus can also be time saving and health promoting—if doing this, get into the habit of *always* looking at ingredient labels to see exactly what is inside the product you are buying.

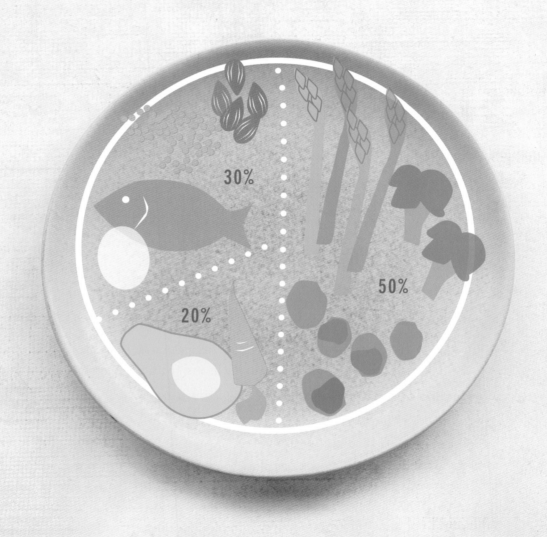

HOW TO DESIGN YOUR PLATE: 50:30:20

Generally speaking, I don't like to be too prescriptive about what exact foods you should be eating and in what combinations. I much prefer you to experiment with wholefoods and find a way of eating that you find enjoyable, satisfying, and sustainable. However, I do recognize that some people will want and need more specific guidance.

For that reason, I have created some simple guidelines to help you get started. A good rule of thumb for eating in a way that promotes health as well as fat loss is what I call the 50:30:20 plate. Don't worry about sticking to these proportions rigidly. They are only meant as a guide.

- **Make up 50 percent of your plate with non-starchy vegetables** such as broccoli, cauliflower, greens, cabbage, spinach, mushrooms, Brussels sprouts, and asparagus.

- **Make up 30 percent of your plate with protein** such as lean meat, fish, eggs, tofu, lentils, beans, and tempeh.

- **Make up the remaining 20 percent of your plate with starchy, wholefood carbs, and/or natural sources of fat**. Examples of wholefood carbs include brown rice and root vegetables (such as sweet potatoes, parsnips, and carrots) and examples of natural fat include nuts, seeds, and avocados.

If you are still feeling hungry 2–3 hours after your meal, I would experiment with increasing either your protein intake, or the overall quantity of food, or both. Some of us, when trying to lose weight, simply do not eat enough at mealtimes, which can result in more snacking later.

If the 50:30:20 plate doesn't appear to be working for you, I've seen people achieve great results with one of the following two tweaks:

- **Reducing natural fat intake and increasing wholefood carbohydrate intake**—meaning they end up with a more "low fat" style of eating. This can work particularly well for people following a vegan or vegetarian diet.

- **Reducing wholefood carbohydrate intake and increasing protein and natural fat intake**—meaning they end up with a more "low carb" style of eating.

I want to make it crystal clear that these guidelines are completely optional. Feel free to ignore them if you don't need them. All of us are different and will thrive on different combinations. Many people can eat wholefoods in proportions quite different from these and still achieve great results. The key to long-term success is to experiment and discover what works best for you and your lifestyle.

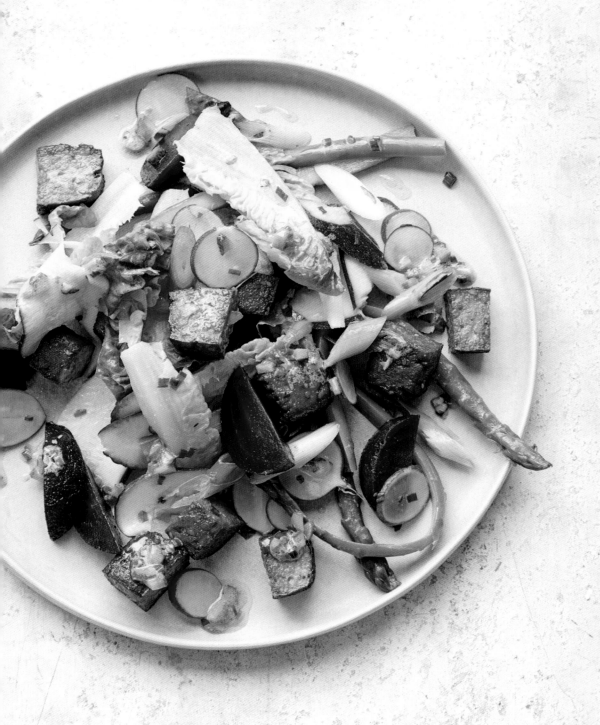

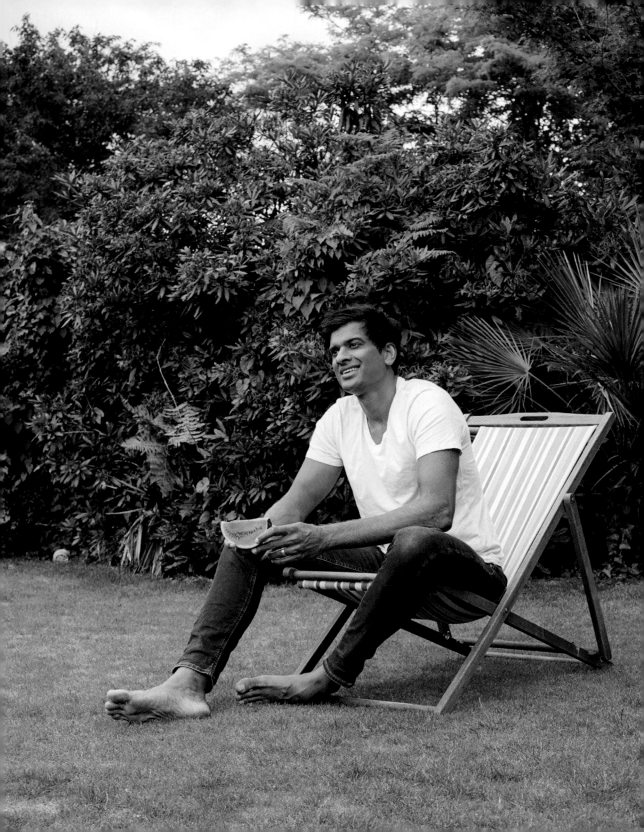

BRINGING IT ALL TOGETHER...

The more you manage to stick to a diet of real food, the better you'll feel and the easier you will find it to lose weight. Not only does real food make fighting hunger and resisting temptation much easier, it also has a huge number of domino effects, such as increased energy, improved mood, and better sleep, which in turn will make every other aspect of your life better.

Here are my top six tips for eating for healthy weight loss. You don't necessarily need to do them all. Experiment, keep an open mind, and, most importantly, have fun!

- **Focus on one-ingredient foods:** Aim to eat foods that are as close to nature as possible. This will help reduce your hunger signals, increase fullness, and nudge your weight point down.

- **Dinner for breakfast:** Prioritize a real-food meal for your first meal of the day. This can have a dramatic impact on your subsequent food choices and increase your energy and improve your mood and focus.

- **Power up with protein:** Ensure adequate protein at every meal. This will help you to stay fuller for longer.

- **Greens go first:** Ensure you have a generous serving of salad or non-starchy vegetables, like broccoli or greens, at the start of each meal. This will help you slow down and eat less.

- **Quench your hunger:** Drink one to two full glasses of water thirty minutes before each meal.

- **Learn to cook:** Being able to cook is a crucial part of moving to a real-food diet. It really does not need to be complicated and I would urge you to learn how to cook five simple meals that you enjoy.

"THE MORE YOU MANAGE TO STICK TO A DIET OF REAL FOOD, THE BETTER YOU'LL FEEL AND THE EASIER YOU WILL FIND IT TO LOSE WEIGHT."

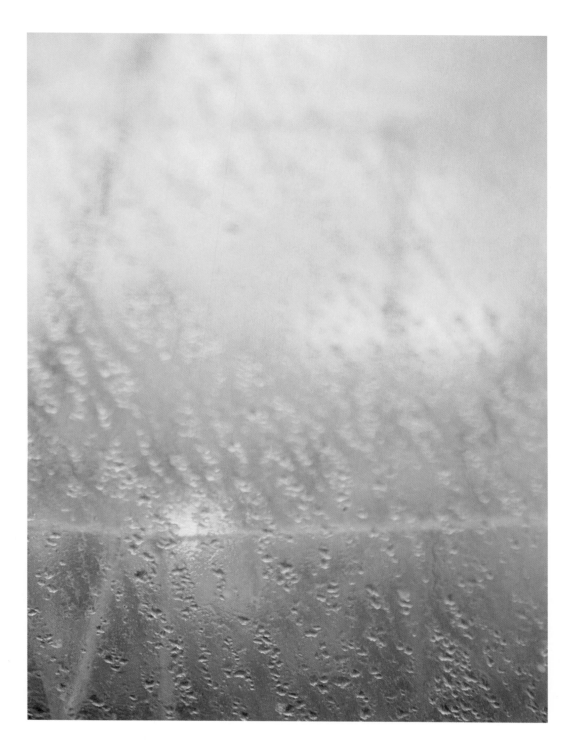

2

WHY

WE

EAT

When we talk about weight loss, we often talk exclusively about food and exercise. We are told that if we want to lose fat, all we need to focus on is the right kind of diet, usually a restrictive one, and the right type of workout, usually a punishing one. This kind of thinking has dominated the conversation around weight loss for decades and not only is it misleading, it's largely unhelpful as well.

There are so many other parts of a person's life that can contribute enormously to their weight—for example emotional problems such as stress, loneliness, and depression. Time and time again, I've seen people who successfully change their diets but are able to lose weight only after they've tackled their stress levels and any emotional factors that were also playing a huge role.

If we are to lose weight and keep it off for good, we need to explore why we're eating too much and why we continue to eat foods that we know are sabotaging our efforts, despite our best intentions. This means going on a journey of self-discovery. I appreciate that this may feel a little bit intimidating but all it really means is that in order to truly change our lives and lose weight, we'll have to get to know ourselves a little better and understand why we've developed a difficult relationship with food in the first place. This means thinking about stress and what's sometimes called "emotional eating;" it means making sure we're sleeping properly, and it means correcting some of the damaging habits and ideas we might have formed around exercise.

This tends to be the area that many people who are trying to lose weight ignore. It's far easier to simply buy a new diet book and follow its instructions. But these books usually don't work in the long term. For many people, this section will be *the* most important. So let's get started.

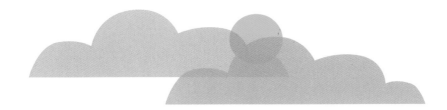

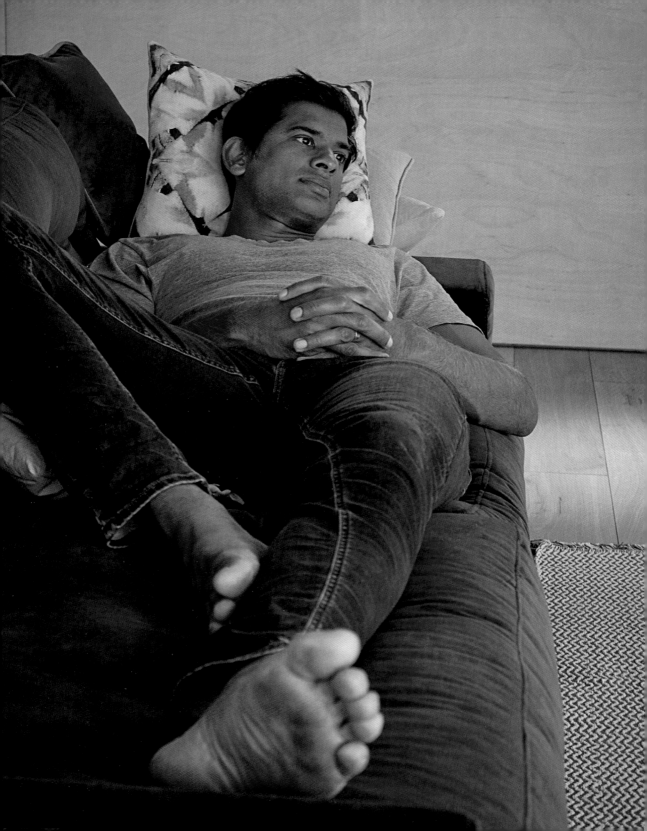

EATING
YOUR
EMOTIONS

One of my favorite quotes is by the famous psychotherapist Viktor Frankl. He wrote: "When a person can't find a deep sense of meaning, they distract themselves with pleasure." I think this tells us so much about our problematic relationship with food. I see it playing out all the time in my clinic. People use food to treat their sadness, their stress, and their loneliness. When their lives feel like they've got a gap in them, for whatever reason, they'll often plug it up with pizza.

I'm sure, from time to time, you've done this. I know I have. When I feel weary and a bit down on myself, I'll sneakily prescribe myself a chocolate bar or something sweet, and do you know what? It will help me feel better— for about ninety seconds. It's the same when I'm on long book tours in unfamiliar countries. When there are no arms around to hug me, I'm regularly tempted to run towards the chemical hug of some blissy foods that are just a friendly room-service dial away.

The crazy thing about this kind of behavior is that my system isn't missing calories but the experience of my wife or children hugging me. I'm not starving for energy, I'm starving for love. Physical contact with my family gives me a natural burst of positive feeling and I get something a bit like that from a portion of ice cream or a chocolate brownie. It's a bowl of warm-and-fuzzies.

LONELINESS

Many people I know eat when they're lonely. Once upon a time, we always ate together. Families and communities would gather at night to enjoy their food as a connected group. When a hunter caught an animal, the meat would be shared. But we're more isolated than ever these days, and researchers know that feelings of severe social separation are rife and rising in the West. If you're feeling lonely, and you don't have those rich, meaningful connections in your life, then that may be why you're spending too much time on the sofa eating cookies and sweets. You feel like you've got a hole in your stomach, but the hole is actually in your heart.

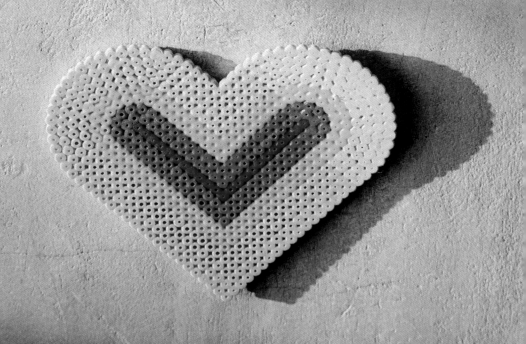

PEER PRESSURE

Some people use food to impress friends and social media followers. We might feel the pressure to regularly prepare meals for ourselves and our families that match up to the gorgeous shots of glistening, colorful plates we see online or in recipe books. Professional content creators have the full-time job of making "healthy" food look perfect and the influencers you're following will likely be among the best in the business. It's so easy to fall into the trap of thinking that's what your meals should look like, too. If you have porridge every day for lunch, or some supermarket fish and a tub of microwaved veggies for dinner, you can feel like you've somehow failed.

SECURITY

Others use food to increase their sense of emotional safety and security. If you're unhappy in your life and feel you have no control over it, you might feel a compulsion to cling on to behaviors you can control. Some people who feel this way end up developing eating disorders like anorexia and bulimia, but many others become overweight. We know that traumatic childhood experiences will often lead to obesity in adulthood, but you don't have to have suffered anything as severe as that to have a problem. If you've had a bad day at work and your boss or team or customers have been knocking you around emotionally, one way of reclaiming your sense of personal control is by deciding to eat whatever you want at the end of the day, and having no one tell you otherwise. That packet of chips on the bus home, or the bar of chocolate in front of Netflix before bed, becomes your act of rebellion, your middle finger to the world around you. You're eating not for fuel but to restore your sense of self-esteem.

CASE STUDY

I first saw Emily when she booked an appointment to talk about her depression. She was hoping I'd prescribe her some medication to treat her low mood, but I was keen to explore her lifestyle to see if there was a way to understand what was at the root of her symptoms and deal with that first. She told me she felt like a "failure" and thought she was "worthless." It soon became clear that a lot of her self-esteem issues were bound up with her weight. She was in her mid-thirties and, over the last decade or so, had been jumping from diet to diet each year. She'd lose a bit of weight, feel good about herself, and then it would pile back on again. Of course, she blamed herself for this.

As we talked, she mentioned her new job, which she hated. She'd only recently moved into the area to take a promotion at head office, and it wasn't working out as she'd imagined. She no longer had a social network, as all her regular friends were far away, where she'd grown up, in South Wales. In the evenings, she felt bored, lonely, and low. This was when she'd sabotage her efforts at losing weight with food. She'd order pizza or devour a large bar of chocolate or a big packet of chips. She couldn't understand why she wasn't able to "restrain" herself and would beat herself up about it, waking every morning feeling terrible inside and out.

I told Emily that I wasn't going to prescribe her antidepressants just yet. I recommended that she phone a friend or member of her family every evening with the aim of really catching up. It only needed to be for a few minutes. If no one was around to talk to, I asked her to join a supportive online group and jump on there to interact and have fun. If, on some evenings, she didn't feel like this, I asked her to do something she really enjoyed that nourished her. She came from a long line of Welsh choral singers on her father's side. She told me she loved to sing but felt embarrassed about it. As she lived alone, I told her to get into the habit of singing one of her favorite tunes after work every day, at the top of her voice.

Over the next few weeks, something remarkable happened. Without thinking about it, Emily started to snack less in the evenings. She was finding it easier to motivate herself to cook nourishing meals, which meant she was eating far less takeout. Cooking was her new relaxing time, where she'd put on a playlist of the tunes she loved and sing them at the top of her voice. It was her new favorite part of the day and, during tough times at work, she would cheer herself up by looking forward to it. After a few weeks, she joined a local choir. This not only gave her a new confidence in her singing talents, but meant she found a new community of supportive friends.

Not only did Emily start feeling good about herself, she started losing weight. She didn't need to rely on blissy foods for a pick-me-up in the evenings when she was having such fun with her new friends. Harsh dieting was never going to be the answer to her weight problems. Once she mended her social connections, she started feeling great and losing weight—effortlessly.

CONNECT EACH DAY WITH ANOTHER HUMAN BEING

Treat yourself with kindness, not with food

Many of us eat to soothe loneliness rather than hunger. This is completely natural and not something to feel guilty about. But if you tend to do this, it will be really helpful to put some thought into exactly what's driving your unhelpful eating habits.

Most people these days would benefit from having more meaningful human connection. One of the simple daily habits my patients have found incredibly powerful is making sure they meaningfully connect with another human each day. Once they make daily connections a priority, they automatically end up eating less and craving snacks less. Even five minutes can be transformative. You could try the suggestions on the opposite page.

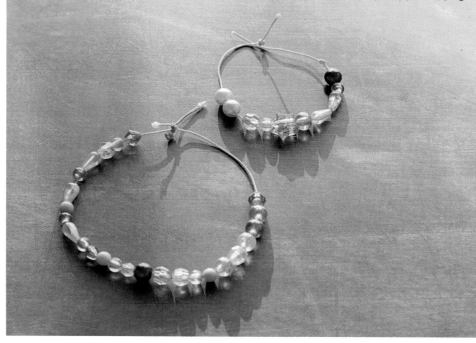

- Phone a friend or family member

- Have a coffee with a coworker and catch up on non work-related news

- If you have a partner or roommate, have dedicated catch-up time each day. Maybe in the evening after dinner, without the distractions of the online world

- Engage in an offline group activity such as yoga, singing, book clubs, Parkrun, or pilates with other like-minded individuals

- Volunteer for a local food bank or charity

- Engage meaningfully with an online support network that has a positive and supportive culture

- Have a chat with your buddies on a WhatsApp group. You could even arrange a set time to do this. I sometimes do this with my friends. We might say, "Let's all jump on at 8 p.m." and for ten minutes we just chat back and forth

- Send a friend or work colleague a voice message telling them how much you value them—and don't expect a reply. Research suggests doing things for other people has lots of psychological benefits

- Share something you find difficult with a friend, family member, or work colleague. Don't be scared to be vulnerable

If you're unable to connect meaningfully with another human being, make sure you connect with yourself by doing something you love, even just for five minutes: dancing, singing, reading, or listening to music or a podcast.

Once you make daily connections a priority, you will find yourself less likely to soothe your emotions with food.

STRESS AND THE STORE-FAT SIGNAL

A couple of years ago, I was visited in my clinic by a woman in her mid-forties called Linda. She and her husband were exactly the same age and also happened to do the same job. They'd met at an insurance company's head office twenty years earlier and both still worked there. They'd spent the seven months since Christmas trying hard to lose weight together. The strange thing was, even though Linda and her husband were eating almost identical diets, he'd been shedding pound after pound, but Linda was struggling.

I asked her about her emotional life. It turned out their young son, James, was being bullied at school. While both parents were, naturally, extremely concerned, Linda had taken it exceptionally hard. She'd been fretting constantly and even losing sleep. I strongly suspected the stress was part of the reason her body was holding on to its excess weight. Sure enough, six months later, when James had been moved to a different school where he seemed to be settling in well, her weight started falling off. Within another six months, she'd overtaken her husband.

There was no way Linda was going to lose her weight until she'd untangled her emotional knot. This is because of the effect her stress was having on her system. The human body has two settings that it moves in and out of, depending on how safe, calm, and secure we feel. We have an action state that prepares us for life's difficult challenges. We also have a rest state that we're supposed to be in whenever life is normal.

The problem is, in our busy modern lives, many of us spend too long in the action state. When we've got lots of deadlines and kids needing to get to school and traffic to battle, we move into this setting. Once we're in action state, the system concentrates its resources on whatever difficulties might be on the way. It gets our hearts pumping and our brains working. It takes its focus away from the digestion of food. It also turns our store-fat signals up, because our body wants to start holding on to as much fuel as it can, keeping plenty in reserve for potentially difficult times ahead.

Over the last few years, a huge amount of scientific research has shone a light on just how bad being in an action state is for our weight. One study, in April 2019, found that when we eat high-calorie food while stressed we gain more weight than if we'd eaten exactly the same thing while relaxed and happy. Not only do we get more calories out of the same food when we're in an action state, it also causes us to change how much we eat. A 2007 report found that an astonishing 79 percent of us alter our food habits when stressed: 43 percent of people ate too much, while 36 percent ate too little.

This is why it's tremendously important to try to eat when we're in a rest state. In reality, few of us do. Think about the times you're rushing out of the door with your two pieces of toast, trying to get it down as you climb into the car. Or when you're in front of your computer with that healthy lunch you put care into making but scarf it down while writing emails or on hold on the phone. Contrast this with having a chilled Sunday lunch. There are no emails to do or kids to run to after-school clubs. You're sitting down with your loved ones, laughing, joking, chatting. When you're in a rest state like this, you're working with your body rather than against it. You'll process your food more efficiently and store less of it as fat.

We all respond differently to stress. Some people stop eating when life is difficult. Their body wants them to keep dealing with whatever's causing the stress, so reduces their hunger signal. For these people, it's fairly ordinary to simply forget to eat a meal. But many who develop a problem with excess weight are the ones who respond to stress by eating too much.

You might remember, when we were discussing the addictive qualities of blissy foods on page 34, that we discovered that the brain learns how to behave with the help of a chemical called dopamine. When we eat blissy foods, dopamine is released. It trains the brain, telling it, "This is what you do when you feel hunger." The more you repeat the cycle of eating blissy foods to stave off hunger, the more often dopamine is released and the more your brain learns the lesson to take you to the fridge or cookie jar whenever you feel peckish. If you eat when you're stressed, it's likely you've trained your brain in exactly the same way. Every time you feel bad, you'll go through this three-step process:

1

TRIGGER:

Feel stressed or anxious

2

BEHAVIOR:

Eat more food (or some other type of behavior!)

3

REWARD:

Feel better

These steps create powerful habits using the brain's reward-based learning system. All of us want the enticing reward of feeling better. We are wired that way. The solution is to do the Freedom Exercise coming up on page 93. First, you identify the trigger, and then your goal is to use a different type of behavior to give yourself the enticing reward that we all want: to feel better.

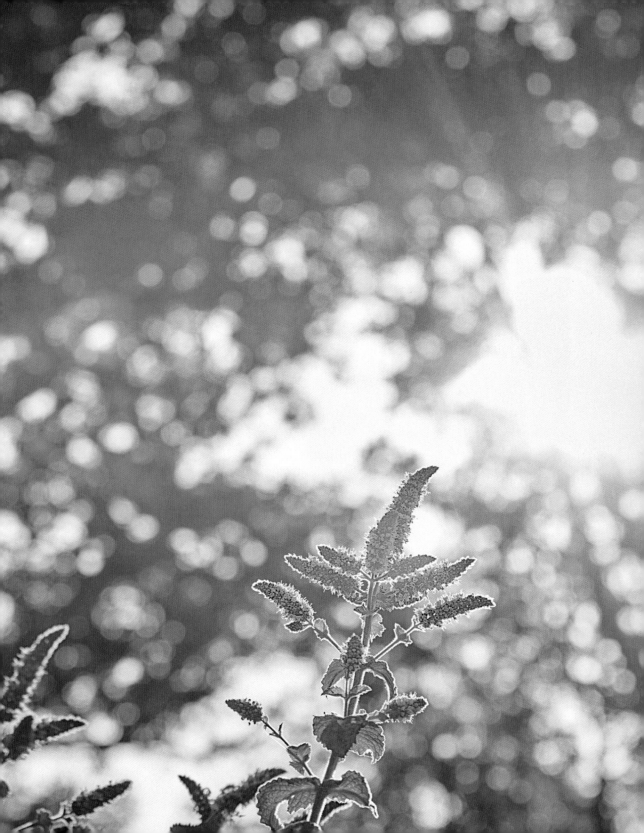

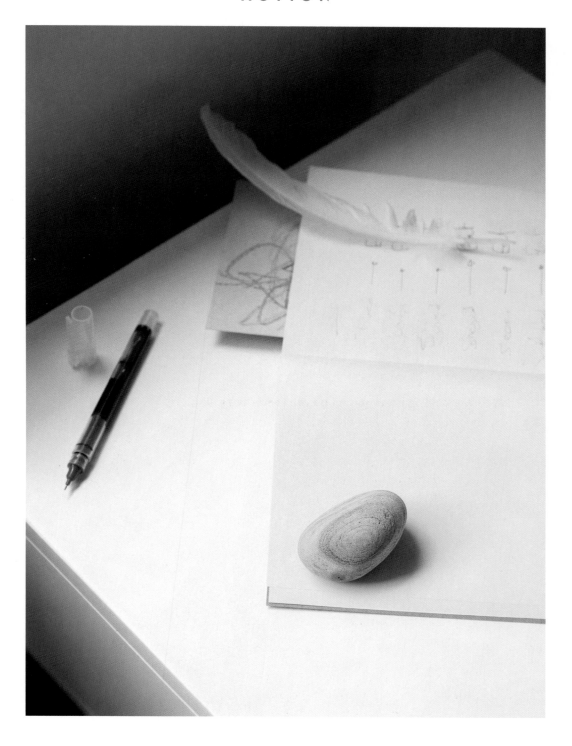

THE FREEDOM EXERCISE (THE 3 Fs)

All behaviors serve us in some way. They are usually attempts to solve problems we're facing or overcome emotions we're feeling. If you're the kind of person who's drawn to food when you're sad, lonely, angry, bored, or stressed, I'd like you to do the following exercise:

FEEL: Write down how you feel the next time you experience a craving
Every time you get a craving, take a pause and try to tune in to what exactly you are feeling. What is the underlying emotion? Is it really hunger or is it something else entirely? Do you feel stressed or lonely? Has something just happened that's made you feel bad or out of control? Do you notice a pattern? For example, does it happen every Wednesday after a stressful and long day at work? Is it after you've had a row with your mother or partner? Is it after a busy day with the kids and a bedtime that's gone on too long? Don't worry if you can't identify the feeling straight away. This will get easier with practice.

FEED: Write down how food helps you feed the feeling
Now that you have identified the feeling, turn your attention to how you try to feed that feeling and resolve the underlying emotion with food. What do you choose to eat? When you consume your chosen food, how does it change the way you feel? Does it make you happier? Does it make you feel calmer? Do you feel less stressed? Or, actually, does the food do nothing to address the underlying feeling—is it simply a distraction? And, if the food does help you, for example, if a chocolate bar improves your mood, how long does it last? Does it completely resolve the underlying emotion or does the feeling of happiness only last a few minutes?

(You may also find it useful to spend some time with the Mindful Moment of Bliss exercise on page 204. This will help you identify the exact point where food satisfies the emotion that you were using it for. You may well find, for example, that one bite was all that was required. Or, you may find that food has done nothing to address the feeling.)

→

FIND: Find a way to deal with the underlying feeling that does not involve food

Next time you feel a difficult emotion that you're tempted to try and resolve with food, why not experiment with some of these effective alternatives instead:

- Try one minute of intense activity such as jumping jacks, push-ups, squats, skipping, or dancing to an upbeat tune that makes you feel good

- Do a relaxing activity, such as yoga, the Five-Finger Breathing Technique (page 96) or meditation, either in silence or using an app such as Calm or Headspace

- Write down how you are feeling on a piece of paper or in a journal. This can be a very powerful exercise to do. Simply giving your feelings a name and seeing them written down is incredibly therapeutic

- Phone a friend, have a chat with someone, or perform an act of kindness, like sending a friend a text telling them how much you value them

- Try taking a short nap, having a shower, or indulging in a relaxing bath

- Try drinking a large glass of water—sparkling can be really effective for many!

- Go to a different room where you don't usually snack—we often get used to certain behaviors in specific environments e.g., eating chips on the sofa

After you have experimented with one of the above options, pay attention to how you feel. Do you still have the craving? Or, has it disappeared?

This Freedom Exercise is about learning and discovering, not blaming and shaming. Be kind to yourself throughout. You are learning to understand yourself better, and what could be more rewarding than that? This exercise, of course, is not exclusive to food. You can use it for any other behavior you are trying to address, for example, drinking alcohol, incessant scrolling on Instagram, or binge watching videos on YouTube.

NB. If you don't have time to do all three steps each time you experience a craving, please don't worry. Even just taking a brief pause to identify the feeling is very helpful. This helps you gain awareness, which is the most important step of all.

ALCOHOL

Drinking alcohol is a classic behavior that many people turn to to help them deal with an underlying emotion, like stress or loneliness, and is frequently the elephant in the room when it comes to weight loss. Make no mistake about it, it's a classic saboteur. It pumps us full of calories that do nothing to stop our hunger signals and in fact often stimulate them, especially after a big night. Lots of us who pay meticulous attention to our diets give ourselves a free pass when it comes to alcohol. If this is you, you might want to gently start asking yourself why. Is it true that the only way to "unwind" or "de-stress" is to have a drink? Or is this the way you've learned to cope with stress?

If you think your cheeky glass of red wine or bottle of beer might be derailing your weight-loss journey, the Freedom Exercise on pages 93–4 can be incredibly useful. Simply substitute the word alcohol for food.

THE FIVE-FINGER BREATHING TECHNIQUE

The brilliant behavioral neuroscientist and psychiatrist Dr. Jud Brewer taught me this fabulously simple technique, which works equally well for adults and kids. It's so great for bringing you back into your body and out of your head in stressful moments—those occasions when you might otherwise head for the cookie jar or the wine bottle. It's magically effective because it uses three different senses: vision, breath, and touch. Your brain can only focus on a limited number of things at once. If you're feeling stressed or anxious and you try this exercise, you'll find that your whole brain capacity is required to perform it, so all that negativity will be pushed out.

1
Hold your left hand out in front of you.

2
Place your right index finger on the outside edge of your left thumb at its base.

3
As you breathe in, trace your right index finger up the side of your left thumb until you get to the tip.

4
Now, breathe out as you move your right index finger down the other side of your left thumb.

5
Continue like this, tracing out each finger in turn, breathing in when going up and breathing out when going down.

You can listen to an insightful conversation that I had with Dr. Jud Brewer about this breathing technique, and other tips to manage your emotions, by listening to my *Feel Better, Live More* podcast at drchatterjee.com/103

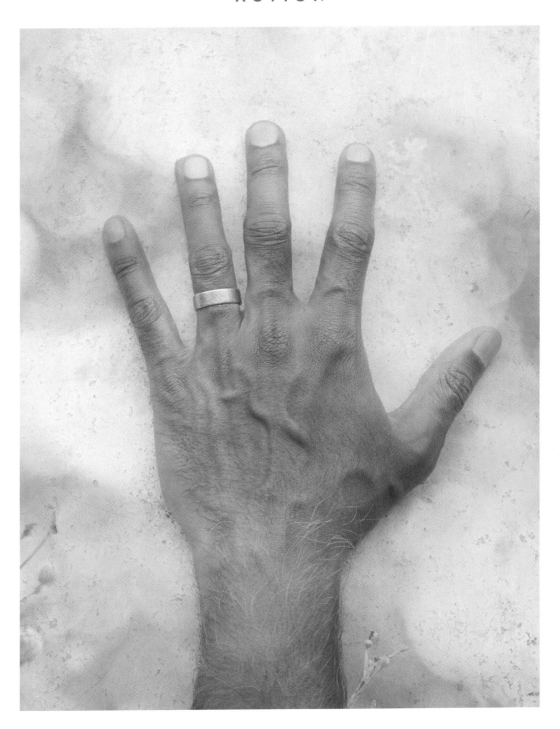

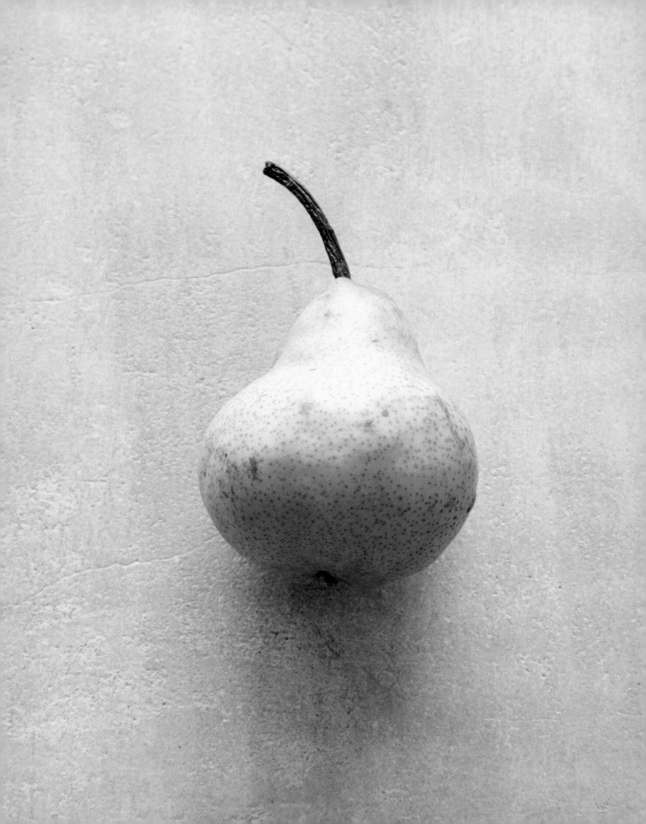

YOU ARE NOT YOUR SHAPE

Many people who struggle with their weight are literally weighed down by layers of emotional baggage that they have accumulated over the years. I have seen many patients in my practice who can't stand to look at themselves in the mirror, because when they do, all they focus on is their size. In fact, some have admitted to me that they hate themselves. If this sounds like you, it's crucial to remember that you are not your shape. Your waist size and your outline do not even begin to define you. You're someone with hundreds of qualities, most of which are far more important than your physical measurements.

If we don't like who we are, we tend to project our negative beliefs about ourselves into the minds of other people. You might think everyone you meet simply sees an overweight person when you walk into the room. This isn't true. Most people, especially your friends, will simply see someone they love and care about, who triggers any number of positive memories and associations. They'll see you for all the ways you really matter to them.

The truth is, you're someone who has found themselves carrying too much fat mostly for reasons you weren't even aware of. Your body has been doing what it's designed to do and responding naturally to the environment it happens to be in. There's no need to shame yourself for how you look. Shame is a toxic emotion that never helps anyone change. It's important that you try to accept yourself as you are and respect the journey you've been on with compassion—but also that you feel empowered. You can change the direction of your journey.

FIXING YOUR SELF-TALK

Say at least three kind things to yourself each day

Do you repeatedly call yourself fat and consider that to be a negative? If you do, you're at risk of defining yourself entirely by your size. All medical organizations that I know of classify obesity as a disease. You wouldn't say "I am ulcerative colitis" or "I am cancer." Nobody ever says that, but they do say it about their weight. This is crucial to get a handle on, because the language you use to describe yourself is more powerful than you might imagine. The way you talk and think about yourself determines a lot of the choices you make. So, how do you talk to yourself about your weight?

If your self-talk is negative, without realizing it, you may be making your weight-loss journey infinitely harder than it needs to be. Think about it. If you constantly tell yourself, "I am fat," in many ways you are defining yourself, solely, by your physical size. Your whole sense of self is wrapped up in those powerful three words, so to lose your fat would be to lose your whole sense of self. I've seen on countless occasions that until people change the way they talk about themselves, sustainable weight loss can feel like a real struggle. So, why not make room for new possibilities that empower you and free you to be whoever you want to be.

I'd like you to say three things in the mirror every morning that are kind about yourself. They can be about your appearance, but they don't have to be. You might find the idea of this slightly embarrassing—but if you do, I believe this is a strong sign that it's an area you need to focus on. It might seem like a small thing, but keeping it going every day will really help to build self-esteem and psychological resilience. You, as a person, will slowly become separate from the excess fat that just happens to be on your body at the moment. This will make it much easier to lose weight sustainably, as it will be less emotionally draining.

To hear more about how powerful the words you use can be, listen to an eye-opening conversation I had with Peter Crone on my *Feel Better, Live More* podcast at drchatterjee.com/121

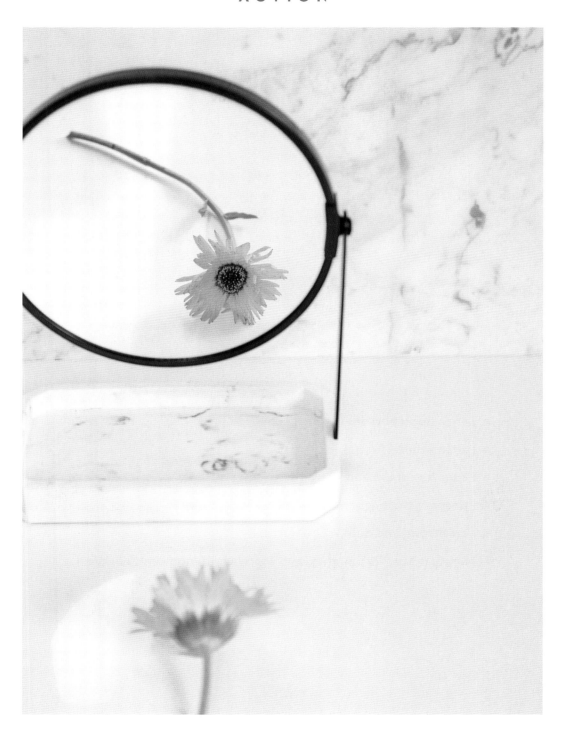

CASE STUDY

Like so many patients who come to see me wanting help with losing excess weight, Candice had a low opinion of herself. Her unhappiness really started in childhood. Candice went to a private school that had quite a harsh bullying culture, and she felt she was constantly being looked down upon because she was on the heavier side. She always felt that if she could only lose weight, everything would slot into place and she could start to live the life of her dreams. She'd spend lots of time in the evening scouring the Web looking for the latest diet hacks, some of which would work in the short term but all of which were impossible to stick with.

I explained to Candice that the only way she was going to lose weight in the long term was to accept herself now. I advised her to start each day in front of the mirror saying three kind things to herself, such as:

- **I am a good person**
- **I am a wonderful friend**
- **I care for others and I care for myself**
- **I deserve the best in life**
- **I am strong and able**
- **I am Candice, I am mighty, and there's nothing I can't handle**

Yes, she found this really hard at first. It's always hard to get over the hump of feeling self-conscious and embarrassed. Before she started, she found it useful to remind herself that nobody was watching her. But day after day, week after week, repeating three kind things to herself daily started to make a difference. She began to feel that she deserved the best in life and that she was strong enough to take on anything the day might throw at her. At work, she stopped accepting it when customers talked down to her. She joined the local yoga class, which she'd wanted to do for years, but had been scared to in case she was judged because of her weight. In short, she started living the life she'd put on hold until she lost weight.

By doing this, she started making better choices. She'd no longer self-loathe in the evening then soothe herself with food. Instead, she subscribed to a YouTube Yoga channel and would do fifteen minutes after work. She also started walking more. These changes led to her sleeping better, which in turn made her feel more confident and empowered the next day. Over the course of a few months, Candice became a new person. Just five minutes in front of the mirror every morning turned out to be the key to unlocking her weight-loss journey. It triggered what I call a "ripple effect," in which one small change triggers the next change and the next change. I see it all the time in my patients, and it can be the cause of health transformations that are almost magical.

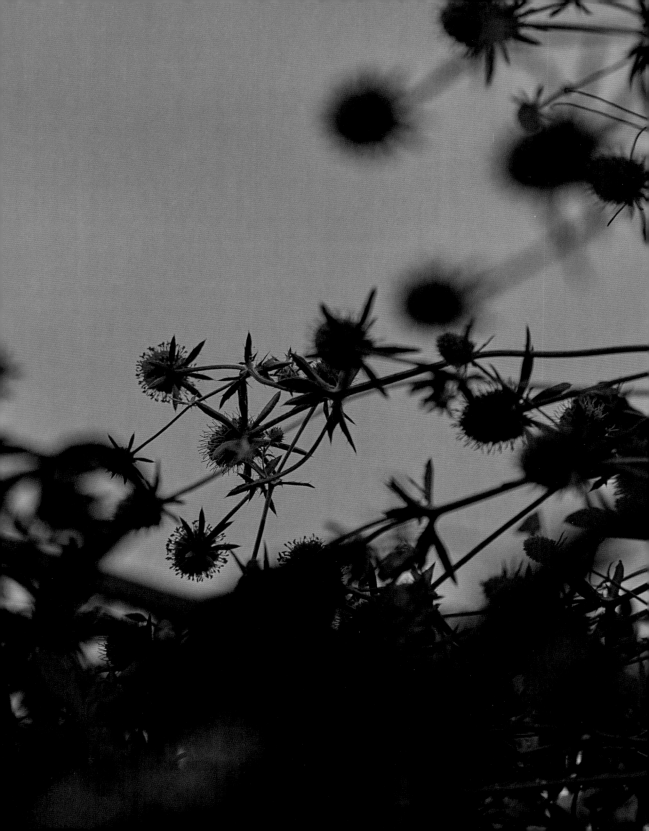

FIX THE UNHELPFUL VOICE IN YOUR HEAD

Our inner language matters more than we think. I'd like you to be really intentional with the words you use on a daily basis. I commonly see the following words and phrases being used by people who struggle with their weight:

- **I can't**
- **I should or I shouldn't**
- **I'm useless**
- **I'm too busy**
- **I'll never . . .**

Without realizing it, this negative self-talk can accumulate over time and lead to feelings of powerlessness, restriction, blame, and guilt.

Instead, I would encourage you to try and swap them out for these empowering substitutes:

- **I choose to or I choose not to**
- **I want to**
- **I can learn how to**
- **I'm not going to make this a priority right now**

Once you get used to using more empowering phrases like these you will feel a greater sense of control and agency over your day-to-day life.

Here are some examples that patients of mine have found helpful:

- **Instead of "I'm too busy to cook a healthy meal"—try instead, "I am not going to make cooking healthy meals a priority right now"**

- **Instead of "I shouldn't have this takeout"—try instead, "I am choosing to have this takeout today"**

- **Instead of "I'm not the type of person who can stick to diets"— try instead, "I've not yet found a sustainable way of eating that nourishes my mind and body"**

It won't be easy to transform your inner language overnight, because you've probably spent a lifetime rehearsing it. But don't let this put you off. Regular practice makes a huge difference. As you start to become more aware of your inner language, you'll soon start to catch yourself when it gets too harsh. You'll also find yourself noticing this kind of self-defeating language in other people. The more you become aware of it, the easier it becomes to change.

OBESITY AS A SYMPTOM

Is your weight helping you on some level? Is there a secret part of you that actually wants you to stay overweight? These might seem like crazy questions, but the human mind is an incredibly powerful organism and can work in surprising ways. One of my patients used to be slim but had become seriously overweight in her late teens. It turned out that her first boyfriend had been abusive. It was during one of her therapy sessions when she came to the realization that she'd unconsciously made the decision that she didn't want to be in a bad relationship again. Something deep inside her felt that putting on weight would stop men wanting to date her. Of course, this is plainly not true, but her brain had decided, without her consciously realizing, that carrying more fat would protect her from danger.

This type of situation is a lot more common than many of us realize. A groundbreaking scientific study led by Dr. Vincent Felitti, the ACE study, showed a strong correlation between people who have suffered from adverse childhood experiences (such as physical and emotional abuse) and obesity. For many people struggling with obesity, their weight is not the actual problem. It's a symptom.

For some, as it was for my patient, the fat that is present on their bodies is there for complex, emotional reasons. But there are other factors at play here as well. As you've already learned, when we feel deep pain, discomfort, and stress, consuming food provides relief and acts as a temporary escape. Food becomes our short-term fix. And what kinds of foods do we crave when we feel like this? Sugar, ice cream, and cakes. There's a reason these foods are called "comfort foods."

If any of the above resonates with you, as well as the Freedom Exercise on page 93, I'd like you to spend some time with the exercise on the next page.

OUT OF THE DARK AND INTO THE LIGHT

Sit down in a quiet place where you won't be disturbed and reflect

Could your subconscious mind be playing a role in your inability to lose excess weight? For example, were you teased as a child and did that make you anxious about meeting new people? Could you therefore subconsciously be holding on to excess weight so that you have a reason not to push yourself out of your comfort zone and make new connections? Or, were you always left out of being picked for sports teams at school? Could you now be holding on to excess weight, so you have a reason to not embark on that new exercise regime that you tell yourself you really want to do? Or, perhaps you enjoy the company and banter with your friends who are also struggling to lose weight and, on some level, you are scared that if you do lose weight successfully, you will also lose the bond you share with them.

There could be any number of reasons playing a role here and my hope is that this exercise starts you off on a journey of self-discovery. Bringing these thoughts out of the dark and into the light can represent a huge step forward in your efforts to lose excess weight and improve your health because without awareness change is impossible.

NB. Some people will require extra help in untangling these deep emotions and will benefit greatly from seeing a qualified health-care professional. If you feel that some deep wounds have been opened up by reading this section, please pick up the phone and make yourself an appointment.

To hear more about how our childhood experiences can affect us as adults, I would urge you to listen to my chat with Dr. Gabor Maté on my *Feel Better, Live More* podcast at drchatterjee.com/37

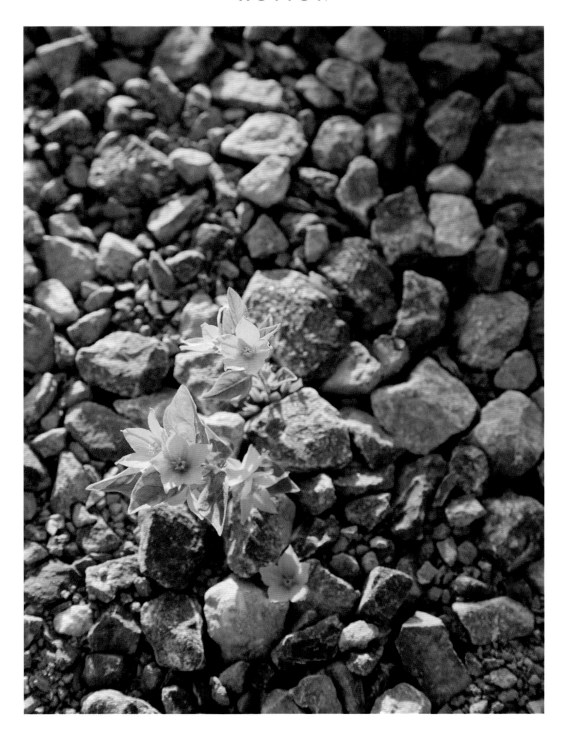

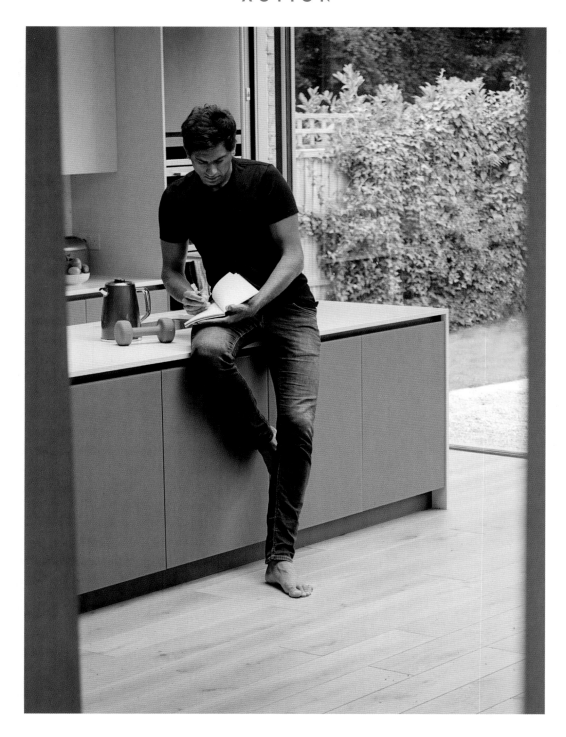

MAKE TIME EACH DAY TO SEE HOW FAR YOU'VE COME

Each day, ask yourself these two simple questions

Getting to know yourself better is an essential component of your weight-loss journey. One of the best ways to do this is to have a daily practice of reflection. If you implement changes to your lifestyle without spending time reflecting, you are missing out on a huge opportunity.

We all sometimes make choices we wish we hadn't. When you do, try your best not to feel bad about them. Instead, see them as an opportunity to learn more about yourself. If you don't take time to acknowledge them and reflect on the reasons you made them, you'll struggle to change your behavior in the long term. Many patients tell me this everyday reflection is one of the most enjoyable parts of their day as they feel they are learning so much about themselves.

I want you to spend a few minutes each day reflecting by asking yourself two simple questions:

- **What went well today?**

- **What can I learn from today and change going forward?**

It's a good idea to experiment with the best time to fit this in so it can become an effortless part of your daily routine. It could be on the commute home after work, after dinner once the kids are in bed or last thing at night. Find a time slot that consistently works well. Make sure you have a pen and paper to hand, in your work bag or next to your bed, as the easier you make it, the more likely it is that you'll do it .

→

Below are some examples that have worked really well with some of my patients and may give you some ideas.

What went well today?

- I slept well last night and have had lots of energy today.

- I had a brilliant day at work and got loads done.

- I was calm and stress-free with my kids after school and enjoyed making them and myself a tasty, nourishing meal.

- I am really pleased with how much I walked today. I walked to work and back, and at lunchtime. I feel great and my mood was better because of it.

What can I learn from today and change going forward?

- I have more energy and crave less sugar when I go to bed earlier, so I'm going to prioritize this tonight.

- I had a bag of chips and a chocolate bar mid-afternoon, even though I am trying not to. On reflection, it was a busy and stressful work day and I didn't have time to take my lunch break. Because I had no lunch with me, I had an energy drink to get me through. Tomorrow, I'll try and make my lunch the night before and take it into work with me.

- I felt really stressed late morning and scarfed down three chocolate cookies to make myself feel better. It worked. Perhaps, tomorrow, I'll try to go for a walk when I feel like that or do two minutes of jumping jacks.

- I made time for a bath last night before bed and the domino effects were incredible. I slept better, craved less sugar, and was less emotionally reactive all day.

"WE USED TO EAT FOOD TO FILL A HOLE IN OUR STOMACH. NOW WE EAT FOOD TO FILL A HOLE IN OUR HEARTS."

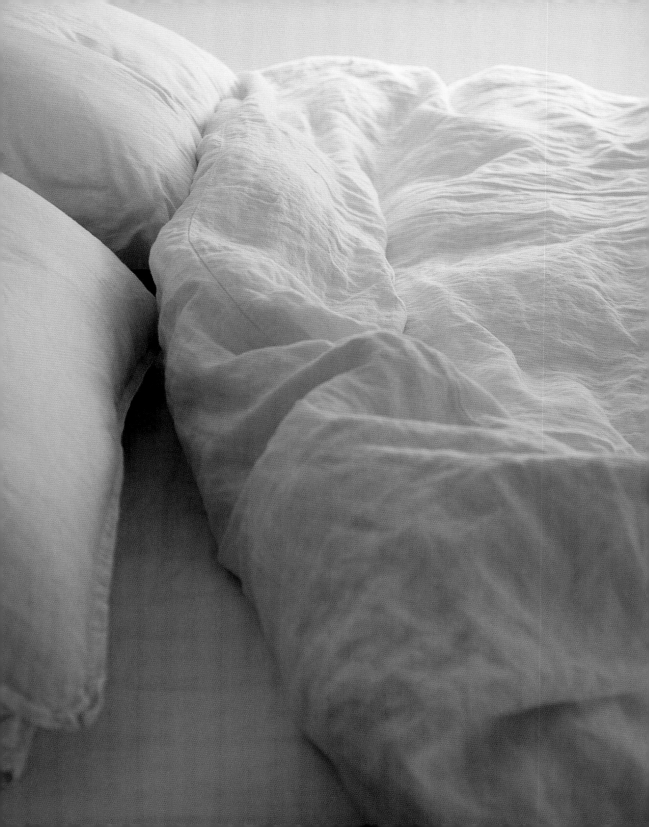

PRIORITIZE SLEEP

After a terrible night's sleep we're not craving fruit and veggies and a cool glass of water from the tap. No chance. We want chocolates and donuts and pastries oozing with cream. You've probably been there, and I know I have. This is why, if you're struggling with excess weight that just won't shift, sleep should be the very first thing you should look at, even before food and exercise. You might feel a little doubtful about this. Surely sleep can't be that important? But the science on this is extremely clear.

Sleep deprivation makes weight gain much more likely. When you haven't slept well, everything else you're trying to achieve becomes much tougher. You'll find it hard to resist tempting foods, you'll be more emotionally reactive, hungrier for less healthy foods, and, when you do eat, it will take you longer to feel full. Starting your weight-loss journey without sorting out your sleep is like trying to juggle while riding a bike. You might succeed, but it'll be a lot harder and will be unlikely to last for long.

A lack of sleep increases:

- **Hunger**
- **Cravings for high-calorie foods**
- **Stress**
- **Anxiety**
- **Emotional reactivity**

HEALTHY SLEEP, HEALTHY SIGNALS

It's really hard to overstate how terrible tiredness is for your hunger and store-fat signals. The science in this area is truly astonishing. One study showed that if you only get five hours' sleep a night, your fullness hormone plummets by 18 percent and the hormone that makes you feel hungry soars by 28 percent. This is a disastrous combination and means, after a bad night's sleep, you're likely to eat approximately 22 percent more calories than you would otherwise. A separate study found sleeping for only four hours leads us to eat about 300 calories extra the next day. Over the course of a week, that's around an entire day's worth of extra calories—just from not sleeping.

Sleep deprivation also increases the desire to choose blissy foods over wholefoods, decreases the body's ability to burn fat, and increases stress, which turns up our store-fat signals. What's more, if we're trying to lose weight when we're sleep deprived, up to 70 percent of the weight we'll lose will come not from fat but from lean muscle, because of sleep's effect on our hormones. And everything gets even worse still if we've drunk alcohol the night before. You may think you sleep especially well after a nightcap or an evening at the bar. However, even though you feel fully zonked out, the quality of your sleep is much worse. We know this from measuring people's brainwaves. After they've enjoyed some wine, beer, or spirits, their brain activity is highly altered. Alcohol sedates us, but sedation is not sleep. Therefore, alcohol before bed can significantly worsen our mood and hunger signals the next day.

I would strongly recommend that you listen to an enlightening conversation I had with the brilliant Professor Matthew Walker on my *Feel Better, Live More* podcast about just how important sleep really is at drchatterjee.com/70

THE CAFFEINE CYCLE

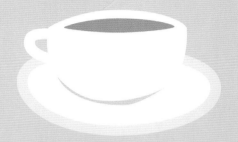

Caffeine is the most popular psychoactive stimulant in the world. And it's addictive. Many people feel they need coffee or tea to keep going, but the truth is, it keeps you in a vicious cycle. Caffeine hangs around in the body for a long time. If you have a large latte at lunch, half its caffeine will still be in your brain at 6 p.m., and one quarter of it will still be active at midnight. This impacts sleep, and that makes you more tired the next day, which in turn means you'll feel more of a need for caffeine to get through the following afternoon. If this sounds like you, I recommend quitting caffeine after lunch for a trial of seven days to see if your sleep quality is improved.

If you are feeling brave, you can even try cutting it out completely for seven days—so many of my patients have tried this and find the quality of their sleep improves immeasurably. Just be warned: caffeine withdrawal is real. You can get headaches, mood swings, fatigue, and so much more, so it can be best to wean yourself off it slowly.

THE BEDTIME JOURNAL

One of the most common causes of poor sleep is having worries and anxieties spinning around in our heads. A simple but highly effective exercise is to simply write down your worries, thoughts, or tomorrow's to-do list on a pad or in a journal just before bed. This will help you feel lighter, calmer, and less anxious, which can be transformative in helping you drift off into deep, relaxing sleep.

If you leave a journal and pen on your bedside table, you'll be visually prompted each night when you enter your bedroom. This will make bedtime journaling much more likely to become an effortless habit.

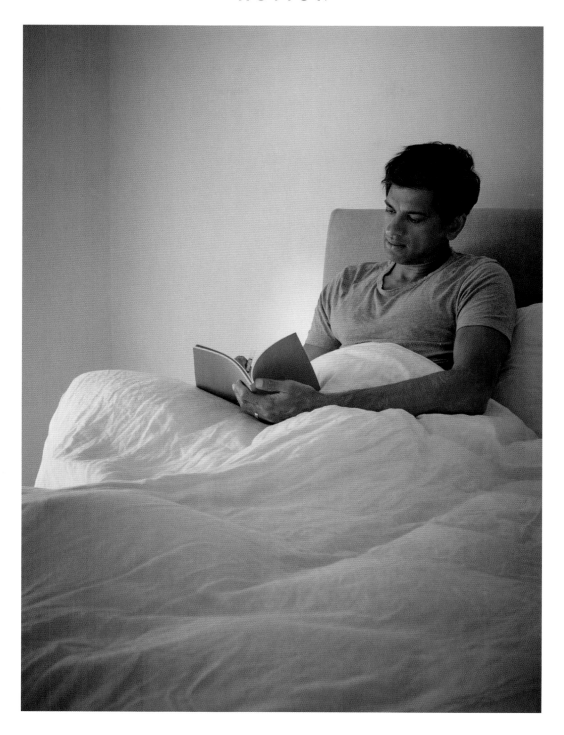

BRIGHTEN YOUR DAYS, DARKEN YOUR NIGHTS

Expose yourself to the right light at the right time

One of the main reasons why so many of us struggle to sleep properly is that we're exposed to too much light in the evenings and not enough light in the day. Our minds and bodies are designed to slowly wind down as the light in the sky changes and day turns to night. A hormone called melatonin helps with this process, spiking in the later hours and helping us to feel sleepy. But artificial light from bulbs and screens plays havoc with this system. Believe it or not, the average person today is exposed to 10,000 times the amount of light at night than they would have been in the 1800s. In the last four decades alone, our exposure to artificial light has increased by 300 percent. When our melatonin system doesn't work as it should, it's not just our sleep that's affected. New evidence suggests it has many effects on our metabolism and digestion, too, and its malfunctioning can increase leptin resistance (see page 42), which means we're less likely to feel full when we eat, and our weight point gets pushed up.

START EARLY ...

The project of getting a good night's sleep starts the moment you wake up. Scientists tell us that high-quality sleep is associated with earlier exposure to bright light in the morning. One 2014 study found that the timing of a person's first bright-light exposure in the day was associated with lower weight. Another found that exposing obese women to at least forty-five minutes of morning light between 6 a.m. and 9 a.m. for three weeks resulted in reduced body fat and appetite.

This is why I'd like you to pop outside as soon as you can in the morning, and look at the sky. Ideally, do some movement or have a hot drink out there. Even on a rainy, overcast day you'll get much more exposure to the natural light your body thrives on than you would in a brightly lit kitchen or office.

... AND STOP EARLY

No less important than getting bright light in the morning is turning it down in the evening. Computers, smartphones, tablets, and TV screens can all emit large amounts of bright light. One study found that looking at a tablet before bed can suppress levels of the sleep hormone melatonin by a whopping 20–30 percent. That's going to have a huge effect on the quality of your sleep, and that, in turn, will affect your weight. Even an e-book makes your melatonin peak later and more weakly compared to a physical book. What's more, a physical book will give you a lovely spike in what's called delta wave activity in your brain, which will help you fall into deep, restorative sleep. (TV screens tend to be less problematic than phones and tablets as they tend to be further away from our eyes, and so the light will have less of a detrimental effect.)

I'd like you to try and switch off all electronic devices (phones, tablets, laptops) at least 60 minutes before bed. If this feels too hard, start small by switching them off 10 minutes before bed and build up from there. If you absolutely "need" to look at a screen before bed, wearing blue light blocking glasses (usually red or amber lenses) can be really helpful.

In the hour before bed it's really important you do something relaxing. Just as children need a bedtime routine, so do adults! Do something that signals to your body that you are winding down and preparing for a deep, relaxing sleep. If you do watch TV, make sure what you are watching is relaxing. Reading a book under a dim light works really well as does some yoga, stretching, listening to music, or a hot bath. Some people, myself included, find it really helpful to do a short breathing practice just before bed. There are many different techniques that work but one of my favorites is the bedtime breathing practice outlined on the next page.

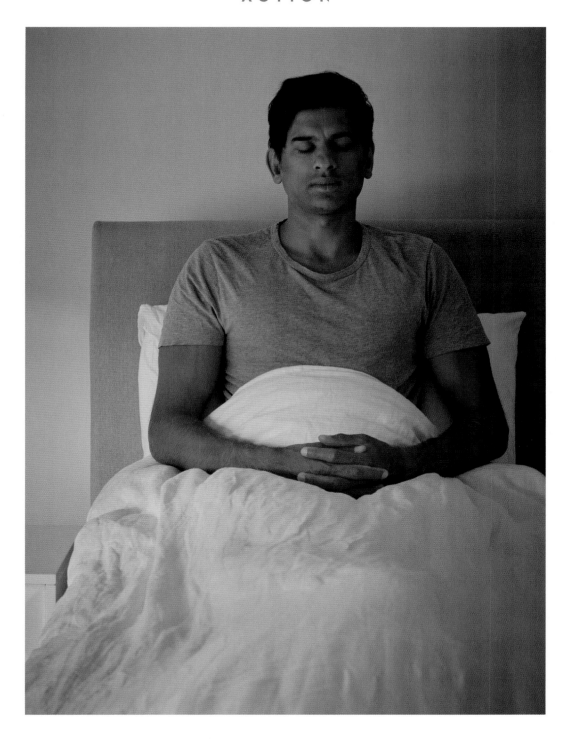

THE BEDTIME BREATHING PRACTICE

This is one of my favorite breathing techniques to practice before bed. I learned it from the brilliant breathing researcher Brian Mackenzie. It's simple, but extremely powerful. When you have a brief pause after inhaling, you help to switch your body into a state of relaxation. Counting your breath also helps redirect your mind away from any anxious thoughts that you might have swimming around.

1

Breathe in through your nose for three seconds (breathing through your mouth is fine, if you are unable to use your nose).

2

Have a brief pause.

3

Breathe out through your nose for six seconds.

4

Repeat.

Repeat this short breathing sequence as many times as required. Sometimes, you may only need to do 1 minute of this practice before you're ready to fall asleep. On other nights, you may be doing it for 5–10 minutes before you start yawning. Experiment and see what works best for you.

For more breathing options, see drchatterjee.com/breathing

CASE STUDY

Sabrina thought she just didn't have the time to lose weight. Not only was her work busy and stressful, she helped care for her elderly parents, who lived with her, one of whom was in the early stages of Parkinson's. There was barely a spare moment in the day to think about food, and plenty of stress and worry, so she found herself living mostly on chips, cheese dippers, and sausage rolls. When I asked about the possibility of her cooking evening meals from scratch with fresh wholefoods, she rolled her eyes. She told me that as soon as she got in from work, all she had time and energy for was to feed her parents quick microwaved ready meals and get them ready for bed.

I asked what she did when they were finally asleep. She told me she cleaned the house and washed the dishes, and by the time she got to bed it was usually after 10 p.m. This is when she'd take some time for herself. She'd either watch YouTube videos or look at Instagram, catching up on the lives of all the influencers she followed. She'd normally fall asleep scrolling and would wake up with her phone under the sheets somewhere, its alarm going off at 5:40 a.m.

It seemed pretty clear to me that Sabrina would find life easier to cope with if she could get more sleep. She readily accepted this, but was extremely dubious about it having any impact on her weight: "How is sleep going to help me lose this?" she asked me, pointing to her hips and belly.

I decided to keep things simple. I asked Sabrina to make sure she got ten to twenty minutes of natural-light exposure every morning. Sometimes, she would sit and have her tea outside in the morning; other times, she'd get off the bus at an earlier stop and walk from there to work. I also asked her to have her last coffee before noon. She had a habit of drinking it all afternoon to get her through the work day, but I explained that this was keeping her locked in a vicious cycle. I also asked her to not take her phone into her bedroom and to buy a cheap alarm clock instead.

Within a week, she was sleeping better. Because she had more energy, she'd walk more in the day. This led to her feeling less stressed at work, so she felt less of a need to stay up late to unwind. She found herself craving less sugary foods and was less emotionally reactive, which made her easier to be around, which made her work life less stressful. Within three weeks, she was feeling able to plan and cook healthy evening meals for herself and her parents.

It was a classic ripple effect, where one small positive change triggers another and another. It did take Sabrina a few weeks, but she started to lose weight slowly, steadily, and effortlessly.

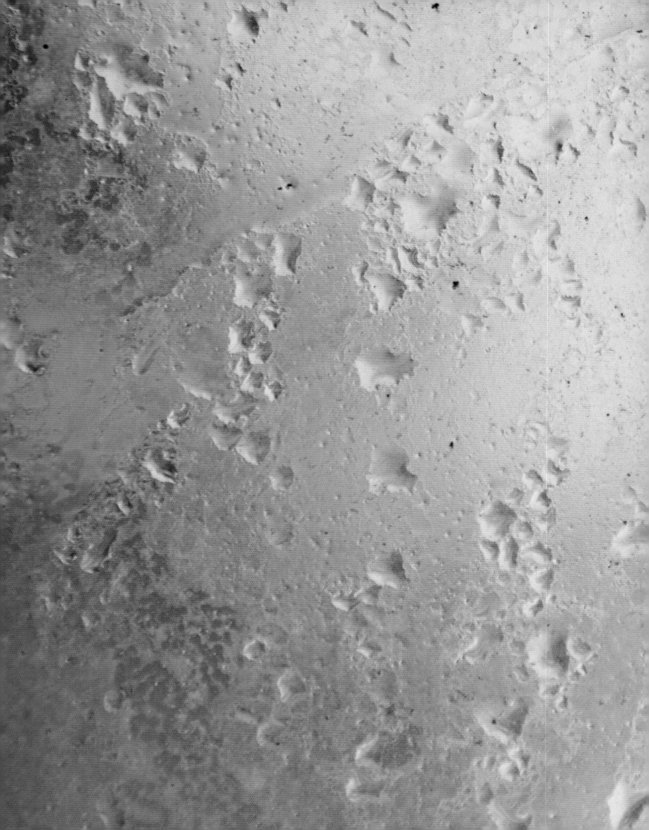

"FOR MANY PEOPLE TRYING TO LOSE WEIGHT, THE FIRST AREA THEY SHOULD FOCUS ON IS SLEEP."

MOVE TO FEEL ALIVE

It's easy, isn't it? You eat what you want and then just exercise to burn it off. If you want to lose excess weight, it's as simple as deciding to eat less and then working up a sweat in the gym. Everyone knows this is true. You've read it in the media, you've seen it online, your friends have told it to you over and over again. It's simply calories in versus calories out. It's so straightforward, so obvious, isn't it?

Wrong. It's actually a lot more complicated than that. While it's technically correct that to lose weight your body must burn off more calories than it takes in, in my clinical experience, using calories in/calories out as a method of keeping off excess weight is generally unhelpful.

For a start, and as we've already discovered, the "calories in" part is extremely hard for you to control. It's actually really difficult to know precisely how many calories any given meal contains, as cooking and processing methods can make a big difference. But, more importantly, hunger is an incredibly powerful, ancient and primal drive. It will always win in the end. If your brain wants you to eat, sooner or later you'll eat. Having the constant willpower to keep your "calories in" down is definitely not the answer to sustainable weight loss.

And "calories out" is even harder to manage than hunger. In fact, it's pretty much impossible. This is because it's not *you* that decides how much energy you're going to burn when you exercise, it's deep systems inside your body that you have little or no control over.

Scientists have discovered that up to 70 percent of what you burn off each day has nothing to do with how many Zumba classes you've taken or how long you have been pounding the treadmill. That 70 percent is taken up with the basic tasks of keeping you alive, keeping your cells working, and your lungs, heart, brain, and other organs going. It also needs to use some of it to keep you alive as you sleep.

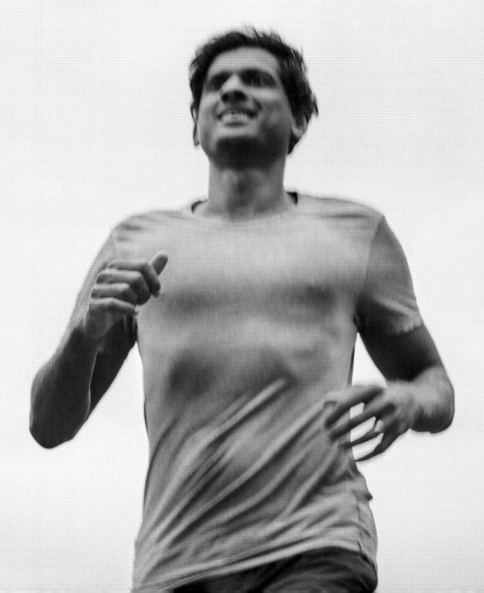

MOVING MORE DOESN'T ALWAYS MEAN BURNING OFF MORE

You might not be surprised to hear that people living in the kind of hunter-gatherer tribes we evolved in have to move around a lot more than the average Westerner, who's often stuck behind a desk or spends their days staring at a screen. You might expect that they also burn a lot more calories, too? Surprisingly, they don't. One study found they burned an average of 2,140 calories per day, which is in a similar range to us. How can this possibly be? Haven't we been told over and over again that we simply need to move more to burn off excess calories?

But those hunter-gatherers are just like us. They're not controlling the "calories out" part of the equation; their bodies are. They're maintaining a healthy weight because their weight points are likely to be set correctly as a result of their simple wholefood diet and their lifestyle. Their bodies have an accurate idea of how much fat they should be carrying and so they effortlessly remain at the right weight.

Your body does the same thing. It tweaks how much energy it's going to burn off in order to keep you at your weight point. If you eat a lot more than you usually would at Sunday lunch, it triggers a series of processes that help burn off the excess calories you've taken in. To take just one example, there's an incredible process that scientists call "non-exercise activity thermogenesis," or NEAT for short. If your system decides you've taken on too much food, NEAT will be activated and your body's spontaneous activity will start to increase. You will fidget more and tap your toes more, without even realizing it. You can't control it. You can't instruct your body to do it more. You don't even know it's happening. It's a completely subconscious process.

To give you an idea how powerful these automatic calorie-burning processes are, consider that the average American ate approximately 500 calories more per day in the year 2000 than they did in 1980. The bariatric surgeon Dr. Andrew Jenkinson has done the calculations on this and shares them in his insightful book, *Why We Eat (Too Much)*. He writes that if Americans are eating 500 calories extra per day, then, in theory, every single year they should put on 57 pounds in weight. In other words, the average American man or woman born in 1975 should weigh more than a ton today! In fact, they only gain around one pound each year. Bodies don't simply take in calories and put on fat—they try to keep you at your weight point.

But these clever processes can become your enemy if you're going on restrictive calories in/calories out-style diets. If you've had a lifetime of blissy foods and crash diets and your weight point has been nudged to a setting that's too high, when you restrict your food your system will fight tooth and nail to get you back to your old weight again. This can affect your ability to lose weight in the long term. So while the underlying idea of calories in/calories out is undoubtedly true—that to lose weight your body must burn off more calories than it takes in—it's so simplistic as to be almost useless as a guide to losing weight.

FORGET THE HEAVY WORKOUT

About ten years ago, a woman in her early forties came to see me in my clinic, having unsuccessfully tried to lose weight for years. She was morbidly obese and yet she'd diligently head to the gym three or four times a week and work that running machine for at least an hour. She told me that she hated it, but that didn't stop her. She kept on going. And yet month after month, for more than two years in all, this woman had hardly lost any weight. In fact, her weight had gone up.

What she didn't realize—and what nobody really knew at the time—was that she was likely to be sending her body powerful signals that were undermining all her efforts. What was happening with this woman was similar to lots of cases I have seen in my clinic. She was exercising too much. Her brain was interpreting these regular periods of extreme stress in the gym as though she was under attack. After all, why else would she be doing it? If she was running that hard and that far, her subconscious system decided, something terrible must be happening to her. So her body was switched into an emergency state. It sent signals that told it to hold on to as much fat as possible. It didn't want to let weight go because it thought, in her place of dire stress and emergency, there was a good chance she was going to need that fat in the future, as fuel to keep her alive.

Heavy, prolonged exercise can sometimes turn the store-fat signal against us. When we're stressed, a chemical called cortisol is released in the blood. Cortisol primes us to get ready for action, making us alert, pumped, and jittery. The problem is, if we're producing too much cortisol for too long a time, it makes our body think that we're in a dangerous environment and that we may not be safe. It wants to store as much fat as possible, for as long as possible, so that it's got it ready for hard times ahead.

On top of that, heavy exercise can have a surprising impact on the number of calories we burn. Conventional wisdom says that when we exercise more, we burn off more—for example, if we burn off 300 calories on the treadmill, then that 300 calories is simply added on to the total amount that we burn off in any given day. Unfortunately, this is not always the case, as our bodies often compensate after heavy exercise—for example, it may subsequently reduce the amount of calories we burn off from processes like NEAT (fidgeting and toe tapping) or make us more tired, so we reduce how much walking and general movement we do for the rest of the day.

In addition, some people find that heavy exercise can dramatically increase the hunger signal. After an hour of aerobics or a blast on the treadmill, they'll find themselves craving large portions of calorie-dense foods. And they have been conditioned by society into thinking that they now "deserve" it, which is why commercial gyms do such a great business in snack foods! Over-exercising in the context of our lifestyle can also affect our ability to sleep, which, as you have already learned, will make sustainable weight loss even harder.

When we do too much exercise, then, not only do some of us end up eating more and fidgeting less, we also store more of the food that we do eat as fat. This is probably what happened to my patient. She fell into a cortisol trap. I advised her to change the way she moved. I suggested that she do a simple five-minute strength workout in her kitchen every morning and aim to walk about 10,000 steps per day. The domino effects were remarkable—

she felt less stressed, her self-esteem improved, and she gained more confidence. This, in turn, translated to better food choices, healthier sleep patterns, less emotional eating, and, ultimately, an enjoyable journey to sustainable weight loss. She started feeling great and, just as I have seen over and over again, this led to her losing weight.

I often think of this woman when I meet people who talk about exercise as if it's a kind of punishment for the sin of eating blissy food. They think that if they work out until they're in lots of pain, they'll have atoned for their crime of eating some chocolate and, having now reset and repented, they've earned the right to have more. This idea is as toxic as it is widespread.

One of my patients has struggled with his weight his whole life. He remembers being on vacation aged eleven and his dad, who also struggled with his weight, took him to the gym. When the boy came off the treadmill and proudly showed his father the calorie counter, his dad said, "Son, you've just burned off 250 calories. You've earned yourself a Mars Bar!" Then off they went to have one. This led to a lifetime of heartache. At no point until I helped him reframe his views did this patient feel exercise was something to be enjoyed.

Of course, I'm not saying that a regime of heavy exercise will never cause you to lose any weight. It quite possibly will, especially in the short term. But if it is going to work in the long term as well, it has to be a regime that you enjoy, makes you feel good, and one that works in harmony with the rest of your lifestyle.

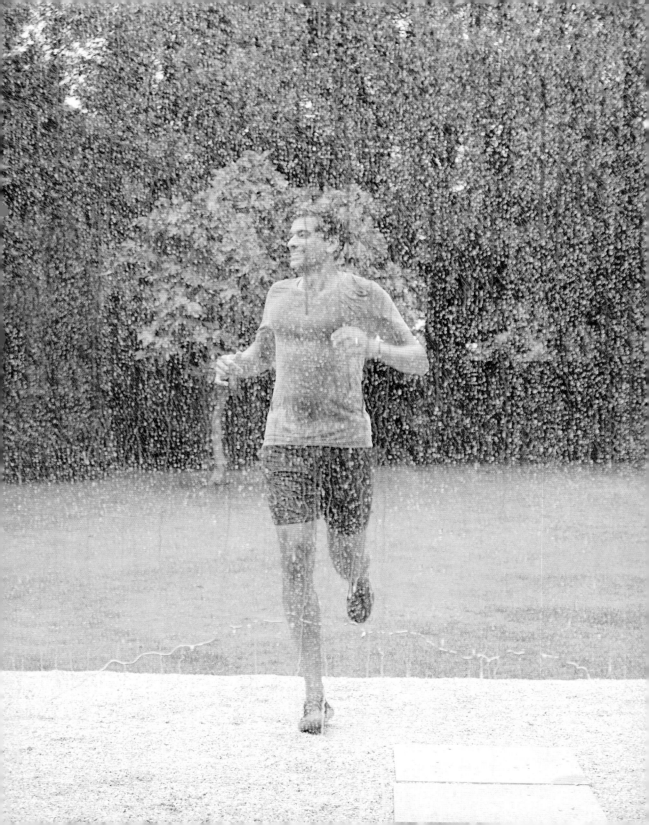

LET'S GET REAL ABOUT EXERCISE

I'd like to help you reset your beliefs around exercise, firstly by changing what you call it. The word "exercise" makes me think of that woman from my clinic, stuck in her cortisol trap, scowling, and in pain. What we're really talking about is *movement*. Movement isn't self-abuse or punishment for a crime, it's a natural and joyful activity that all bodies want to do. Movement is fundamental to who we are as humans. To speak is the movement of your jaw. To breathe is the movement of your lungs. To walk is the movement of your muscles. Movement is life. It really is that simple.

Yes, it's true, increasing movement *might* help you burn off some extra calories. But that's not the main reason I'd like you to do it. This may sound controversial and in conflict with everything you've ever heard before about weight loss. But here it is.

I don't want you to move to burn more calories or to earn yourself a chocolate bar. I want you to move to feel good about yourself: to feel strong, to feel powerful, and to send your body the signal that you're alive and that you're worth it. Self-esteem is one of the most important yet undervalued factors in achieving sustainable weight loss. If you have a low opinion of yourself, or constantly feel guilty for the choices that you've made, you're likely to find it much harder.

So forget exercise. If this is a surprising sentence to read in a health book, it's probably because there's a multibillion-dollar industry set up around the idea that movement is separate from your everyday life. We're told you have to buy the products, wear special clothes, pay for the class. Some of us are more bothered about looking fit than actually being fit. I believe we're making "exercise" too hard. We're overcomplicating it. As the esteemed obesity researcher and author of the brilliant book *The Hungry Brain* wrote: "Our distant ancestors had a word for exercise: life." Look at wild animals and how they move, compared to the average day in modern human life, all of us caged into offices, trains, cars, and lounges. We're animals, too, and it's fundamental to our wellbeing that we move.

SMALL CHANGES, BIG RESULTS

Can you really lose weight without doing any planned movement at all? Yes, you absolutely can. But you might find yourself struggling over the longer term. Habits of movement are critical to maintaining a healthy weight because of the effect they have on your body's signals. Small doses of daily movement signal to your body that you're an active, thriving human and, over time, this will help lower your weight point, which means you'll start to lose fat without really trying. So forget working out for an hour, three times a week—unless you do that already and enjoy it. This is about manageable and regular bite-sized habits of movement.

I'd like you to start small and do the same things every day. If you get into the habit of moving regularly, even for just five minutes, you'll quickly notice changes in how you feel about yourself. These changes to your self-image are just as important—I'd argue even more important—than the changes they'll make to your body. Right now, you might have the identity of someone who can't lose weight. Someone who has failed. By regularly moving and getting your heart pumping, you'll start to take on the identity of someone who chooses to prioritize their physical wellbeing. You'll take on the identity of someone healthy. You'll start to feel good about yourself, which, in turn, will help you lose excess weight.

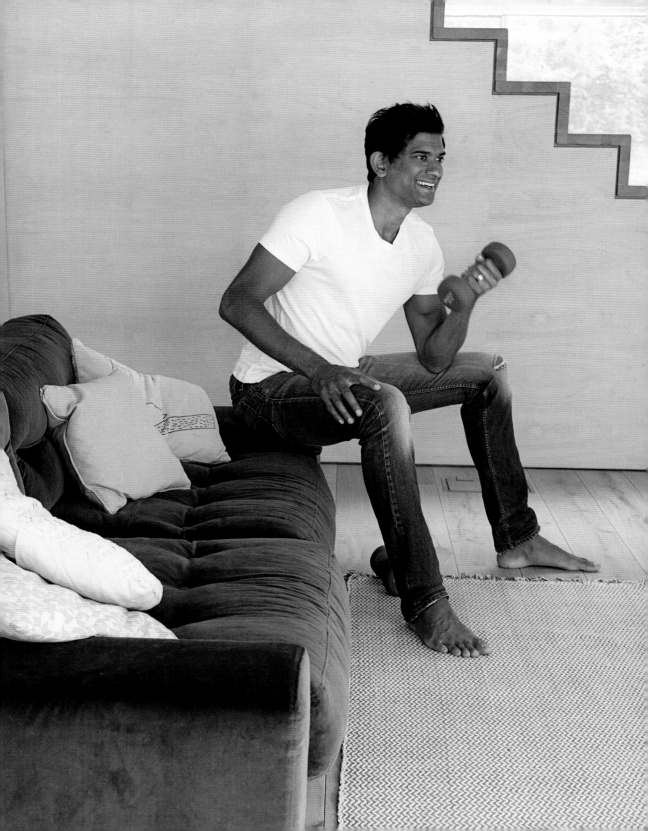

THE SPECIAL CASE FOR STRENGTH

One side effect of our obsession with sweating and suffering is that we've overly focused on aerobic exercises like running and cycling and neglected strength training. To be clear, there is nothing wrong with running and cycling and, of course, they can provide many benefits, but there's something so satisfying about lifting weights. The feeling you get afterwards is unique. You feel strong. You feel more confident. And, with a little bit of time, you start to see changes in your physique.

And, don't worry, this isn't about having a beach body for July or looking like a bodybuilder; putting on that amount of bulk is actually very hard. It's about getting your body and its hunger and store-fat signals working properly. It's also about self-esteem. Nobody ever felt worse about themselves after lifting some weights.

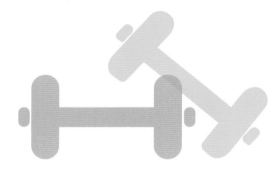

When it comes to fat loss, strength training has some unique benefits:

- **It helps to increase lean muscle mass.** This gives the body extra room to store fuel that would otherwise be turned into fat.

- **It helps your body to burn more calories,** even after the workout is over. This is because the more muscle mass you have, the more fuel your body needs to keep you going. This makes sustainable weight loss much easier.

- **It helps your insulin system work better,** which turns your store-fat signals down.

- **It doesn't tend to increase the hunger signal** as much as endurance-type exercises, such as running and jogging. Over time, this can result in you craving less food, which, of course, will help you lose weight.

I think that we've made the idea of strength training far too complicated. You don't have to join a gym or buy special clothes. Our ancestors didn't lift heavy objects at scheduled times every Monday, Wednesday, and Friday. Simply doing a few minutes each day can rapidly build self-esteem and muscle mass, and it can easily be done in the comfort of your home. I'd like strength-based movement to form part of your identity and for you to send your body a daily signal that you're someone who prioritizes your health. It's consistency, not intensity, that's most important.

MAKING NEW HABITS IS EASY (AND NEEDS TO BE EASY!)

I'm lucky enough to have become friends with, arguably, the world's leading expert in human behavior, Professor B. J. Fogg. He's spent his professional life studying this topic and has found that, in order for us to carry out any given behavior three different things need to come together at the same time: motivation, ability, and trigger.

- **Motivation**: how motivated are we to do the behavior?
- **Ability**: how easy is the behavior to do?
- **Trigger**: what will trigger us to do the behavior?

The secret to creating new habits is to understand how to manipulate these three things effectively. If your motivation is high, you will do things that are hard to do. When your motivation is low, however, you will only do a behavior if it is easy to do. Just think about all the people who stick to grueling fitness regimes at the start of January each year when their motivation is high, only to find themselves back where they started by the end of the month, when their motivation has dropped.

If your movement session is easy and quick and doesn't involve any messing around with traveling to a gym or putting on special clothes, you're much more likely to get it done, even when your motivation plummets. And, remember, your motivation will always plummet!

The final piece of the puzzle is the trigger. Every single human behavior requires a trigger. A trigger might be your memory—you simply remember to do the behavior that you are trying to start. While this trigger does indeed work, it just happens to be very unreliable! The very best trigger is to stick your new behavior on to a habit you already have. That means sticking it on to a behavior that you already do without even thinking about it. This might be straight after brushing your teeth or after boiling the kettle. Or, it could be last thing at night when you get into your bed. The key is to find out what works best for you.

I firmly believe that the kitchen is the very best place to work out because it is a room that all of us visit on a daily basis. For years, I have advised many of my patients to put a dumb-bell or kettlebell in their kitchen and to make it a rule that they won't have their mug of coffee or tea (or breakfast!) until they've lifted. Even if it's just one bicep curl!

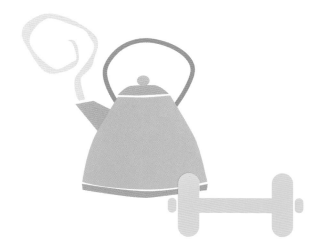

CELEBRATE YOURSELF

Whenever you complete a movement session, it's important to allow yourself to feel fantastic about yourself. Positive emotion is a powerful signal that tells you to repeat a behavior. Please do not be tempted to skip this step. Professor B. J. Fogg's research has shown that these positive emotions help to lock in the new behaviors much more effectively than simple repetition.

Some people find wall charts on which every successful day is ticked off extremely powerful. They can help build momentum and self-esteem. It's intensely satisfying to look at a row of check marks, which in turn motivates you to move more so that you can add more check marks. Some of my patients like to fill glass jars with beans or coins, so they can easily see a visual record of how much they've done. Others like to celebrate when they've finished each movement by shouting things like, "Yes!" or "I love moving my body!" This might sound embarrassing, but you can do it quietly if you need to. The most important thing is to give yourself a shot of positivity every time you do some planned movement. Give yourself permission to feel amazing.

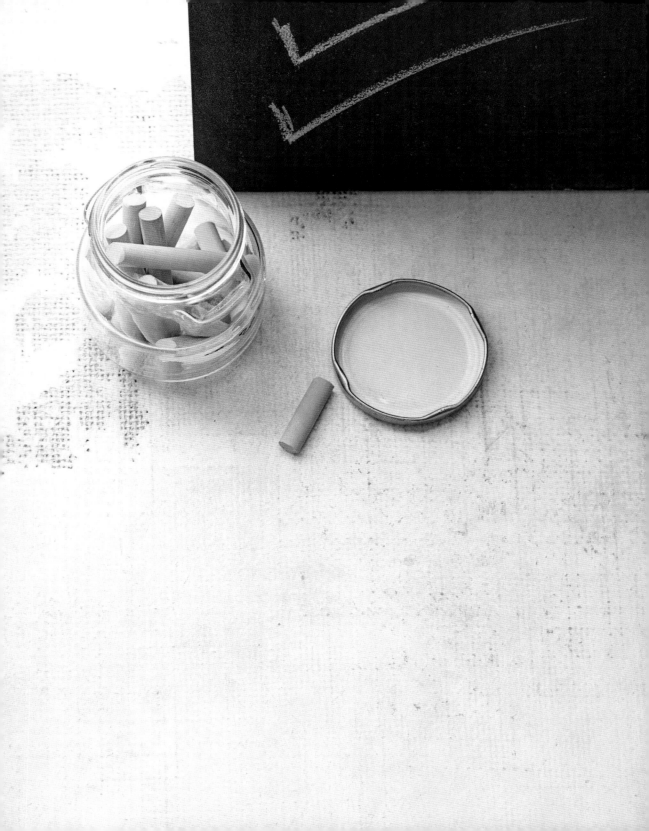

LIFT SOMETHING EVERY DAY

Lift some weights before enjoying your morning beverage

I want you to lift something every single day. Start with five bicep curls a day on each arm, then build up from there. Bicep curls are one of the simplest exercises to get started with as they are easy to do and have a low risk of injury.

Stand up or sit down with a dumb-bell in your hand, ensuring your back is straight. Bring the dumb-bell up to your shoulder using a curling motion. As you are doing this, keep your elbow close to the side of your body. Then return to the starting position. Pick a weight with which you can comfortably do five curls and make sure you do both arms.

Keep your weights somewhere convenient and highly visible so you are constantly being prompted to pick them up. If you keep them out of sight in a cupboard, you will be less likely to lift them. If you feel this will be an eyesore, let me ask you something. How important is it to you that you lose weight? Is it more important that the weight is put away in a cupboard or is it more important that you do a daily habit that will make you feel good, feel strong and, ultimately, more likely to lose weight for good?

I have seen the amazing benefits of creating this simple habit, with thousands of patients. It's so easy to get into the habit of curling some weights every time the kettle is boiling. After a few days, you'll actually start to crave the feeling of your muscles being stretched, as well as the feelings of positivity and joy that you will experience afterwards.

Over time, you can experiment with higher repetitions, heavier weights, and different exercises. On some days, five biceps curls is all you will do, and that is completely fine. On other days, however, you may do a full five-minute workout. The key to long-term success is to make sure you do something each day, no matter how small.

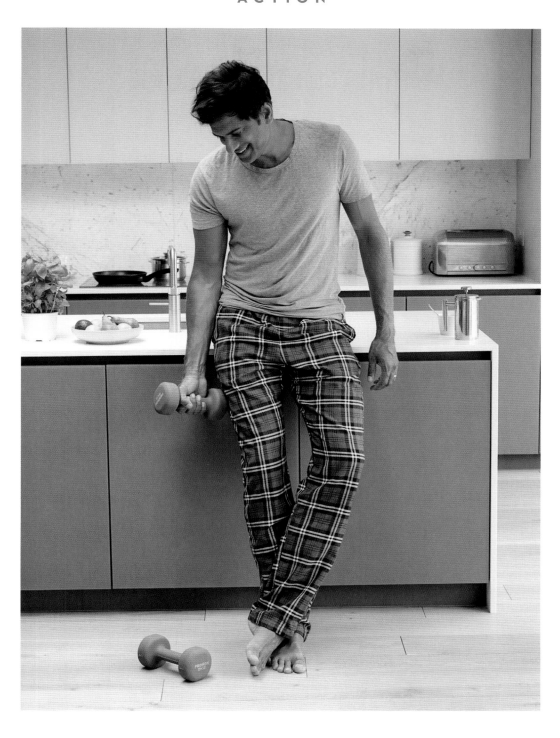

FIVE MINUTES EACH MORNING ...

Over time, I would encourage you to build up to five-minute workouts each day. I have been doing five-minute strength workouts every morning for years, while my coffee brews. This is not because I am more motivated or have more willpower than you. It's simply because I have implemented the principles of successful behavior change that I outlined above. I have made it easy to do, I stick it on to an existing habit and I take a moment to feel good about myself once I am done. There is no reason why you can't build this habit into your life just as easily!

I am a big fan of body-weight movements, like push-ups and dips, because they don't require any equipment. However, I have found that many of my patients, particularly those who are trying to lose excess body fat, prefer to start with something like a dumb-bell or a kettlebell. It can often feel less daunting and easier to get started. If you have one lying around at home, great; if not, you can usually pick one up for under $10 online.

(If you don't want to purchase weights or if you prefer to focus on body-weight movements, you can see some videos I have made to help you get started at drchatterjee.com/bodyweight.)

THE CORE KITCHEN THREE

I have designed a simple routine consisting of only three movements that has the optimal blend of ease and effectiveness. They are perfect to do every morning before breakfast, each time you go into your kitchen, or even every time you make your coffee!

THE THREE COMPONENTS ARE:

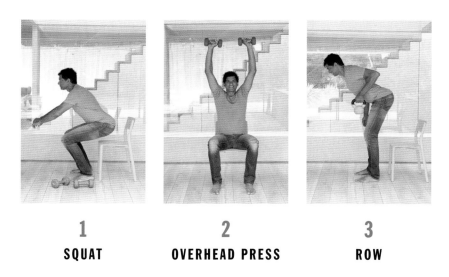

1	2	3
SQUAT	OVERHEAD PRESS	ROW

Feel free to experiment and change it up as you see fit, and don't forget to take a moment to acknowledge how great you feel at the end!

1
SQUAT

Squats are a core movement pattern that we require for everyday life, whether it be to go up stairs or to get in and out of chairs.

Stand with your feet slightly turned out and a little wider than hip width apart. Lower your body towards the floor, as if you are sitting down. You can put a chair behind you and sit down on to it if you wish. This can help build up your confidence. You can also hold on to a wall or a table to help with balance if you need to.

As you go down, keep your back straight and your chest facing the wall in front of you. It can be helpful to look straight ahead of you rather than at the floor below. Try and ensure that your knees are following the line of your feet as you go down. Aim to go down until your thighs are parallel to the floor. Then squeeze your bottom muscles tightly and return back to the starting position. Aim to repeat five to ten times.

As soon as you feel ready, move up to performing squats with dumb-bells, kettlebells—even cans of beans—in each hand.

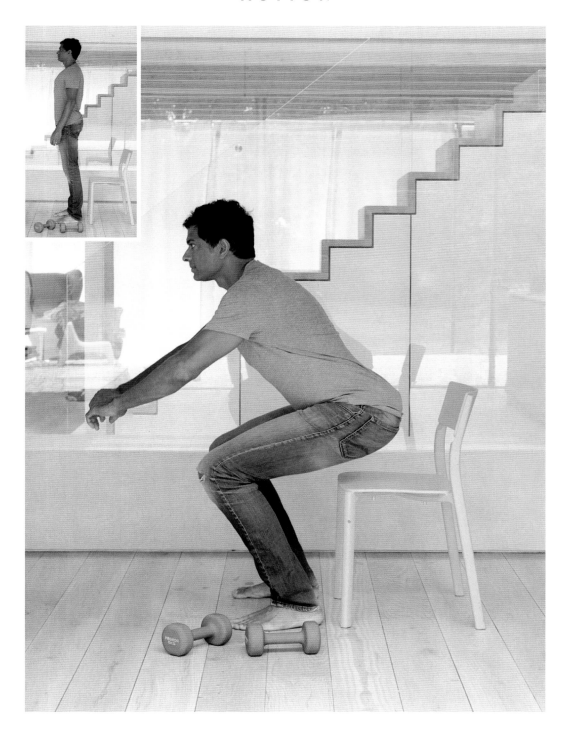

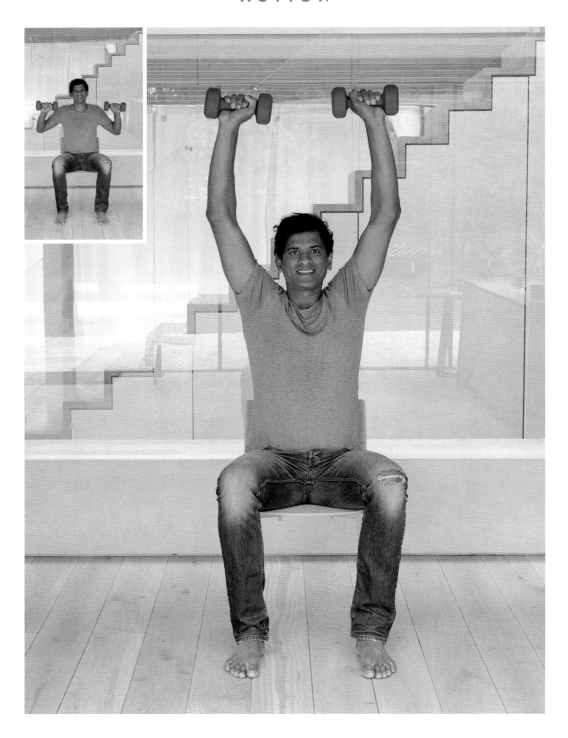

2
OVERHEAD PRESS

Either sitting in a chair or while standing, push both dumb-bells or a kettlebell straight overhead towards the ceiling. Make sure you keep your tummy muscles engaged and your back straight. Try not to poke your head forward as you raise the weight. Then return the weights to the starting position. Aim to repeat five to ten times.

If you only have one kettlebell or dumb-bell, you can do one arm at a time. Make sure you do equal amounts of repetitions on both sides.

3
ROW

From standing, hinge forward at the waist, keeping your back straight and a slight bend in both knees. Hold the kettlebell or dumb-bell in your left hand. Keeping your tummy muscles tensed, pull your left elbow up towards the ceiling until it reaches just behind your back. You'll feel your upper-back muscles contract at this point. Keep your elbows tight to your body rather than poking out at the side. Now lower the weight back to the starting position in a controlled manner. Repeat five to ten times on each side.

If you have two dumb-bells or two kettlebells, you can do both sides at the same time, which reduces the time taken by half so is perfect if you are pushed for time!

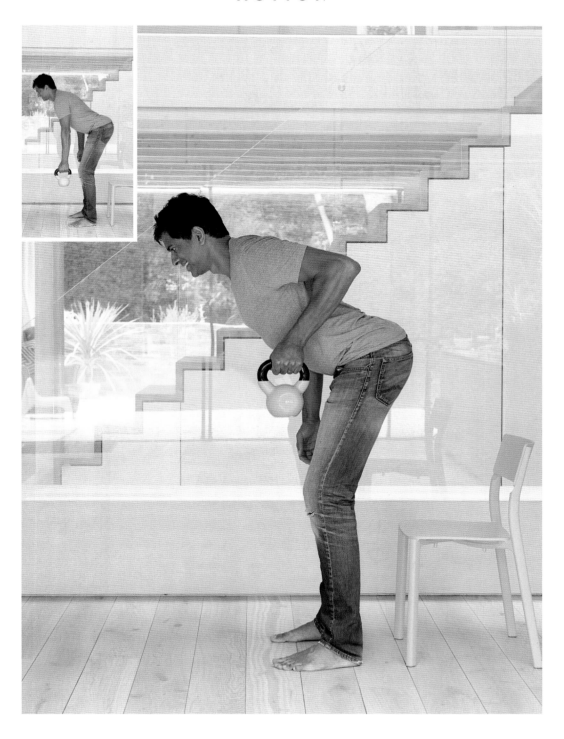

CASE STUDY

Amol wanted advice on his exercise regime. For the last few months, he'd been hitting it hard with four one-hour sessions per week with his personal trainer. But he'd hit a plateau with his weight loss and wanted to find out from me how he could push himself even harder.

It sounded to me like he was pushing himself hard enough. So I decided to delve into his lifestyle and see what I could discover. He told me straight away that he'd eat a lot in the evenings, especially after he'd been killing himself in the park with his PT. He felt he'd deserved his extra calorie load and, as it was mostly in the form of "healthy" protein bars, thought it was appropriate. He also mentioned in passing that he'd struggle to get to sleep after he'd been working out.

I persuaded Amol to experiment with dropping his PT sessions completely, just for a month. Instead, while his kettle was boiling in the morning, he was to do five to ten bicep curls on each arm with a light dumb-bell that he'd keep by his toaster. It took under 30 seconds to do! Once he got used to this, he quickly progressed to doing five minutes of strength work each morning. Straight away, his sleep improved and he stopped gorging on protein bars four times a day. To his astonishment, stopping his PT sessions didn't cause him to add on any fat at all and he found himself with more energy. He started to walk to work. Then he made it a rule that he'd leave the car at home for every journey that took less than forty minutes by foot. Meanwhile, in the kitchen, he was able to lift heavier and heavier weights, and lift them more frequently.

It took just over three weeks, but Amol eventually broke through his weight-loss plateau. He was amazed to discover the answer to his weight problems hadn't been pushing himself harder. Instead, by fitting in small doses of regular movement around his life, and making it an ordinary, non-stressful part of his routine, he got to his ideal size. And he saved a lot of money too.

MAKE WALKING YOUR DEFAULT

As well as lifting something heavy each day, I would like you to focus on arguably the most undervalued movement of all: walking. It's such a beautifully human thing to do and our bodies are highly specialized to do it. In fact, some researchers believe we evolved to walk as many as 20 miles a day, right up to old age. Once upon a time, walking was essential for our survival. It allowed us to hunt, capture prey, and bring it back home to be cooked. Other large animals just can't do this. They're able to run quickly in short bursts or leap from tree to tree, but none are as brilliant as we are at simply putting one foot in front of the other—and then keeping going.

Increasing the amount of time you spend walking can have hugely beneficial effects on the mind and body. Every time we walk, we release special molecules into our bloodstream called myokines, which can make us more resistant to stress and help our store-fat signals work properly. Research shows that just thirty to forty-five minutes of brisk walking per day is enough to provide all the benefits for general health and longevity. This is why I want you to walk as much as you possibly can. In fact, I'd like you to make it your default.

This means seeking out every opportunity you can to walk: using foot power to get you to the shops, school, and workplace, and taking the stairs, not the escalator or elevator. When this isn't possible, see how much walking you can add into your journey. If you park an extra ten minutes from school, in the morning and afternoon, that's over an hour and a half extra walking you'll do in just one week. And remember, this isn't about calories out. Forget calories: think signals. Walking several times each day, even if for a short period, will send your body a daily signal that you're a thriving human being engaging in an active life. When was the last time you went for a walk and came back feeling worse?

WALK EVERYWHERE

I want you to take every opportunity you can to walk. Aiming for 10,000 steps per day is a great target for most people but don't get disheartened if you don't reach this number. Anything is better than nothing. It's just a matter of consistency and steady progress.

Track how much you currently walk, on a smartphone or smartwatch if you like, and see if you can make small, regular improvements. If you prefer not to use technology (like me), simply aim for around forty-five minutes each day, and remember you don't have to do it all in one go!

- Consider walking to work, school, or the shops
- Get off the bus a few stops early or park farther away
- Try a quick five-to-ten minute walk before breakfast or go up and down your stairs a few times
- Walk fifteen minutes every lunchtime (in nature, if possible)
- Try a quick walk around the block before dinner and/or after dinner
- Try standing when using public transport
- Consider joining a local walking group or schedule regular walks with friends as a way of catching up

While walking, try not to be constantly looking at your phone. Try and enjoy the experience and pay attention to how you feel. Once you have finished, take a few moments to pay attention to how you felt, before, during, and after. You may have more energy, feel in a better mood, feel more positive about the world or have solved a problem you had previously struggled to solve. The more you can become aware of these positive feelings, the more motivated you will be to keep engaging with them.

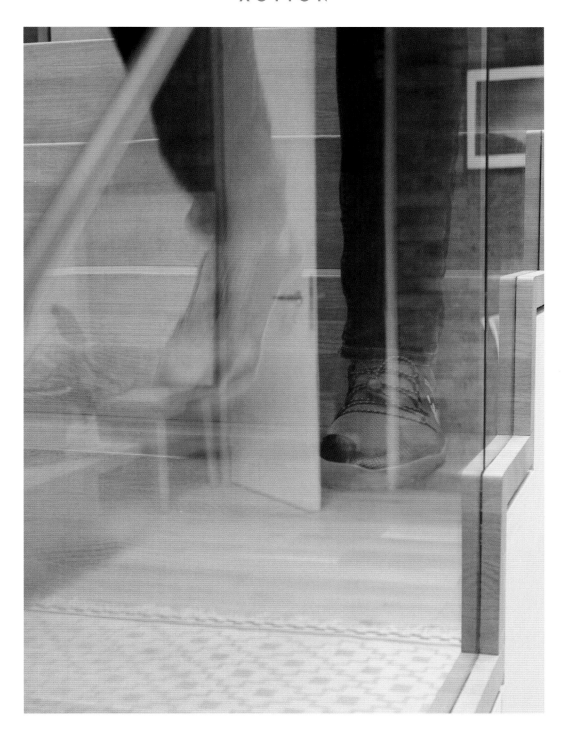

EMBRACE ENJOYABLE MOVEMENT

Although the main goal with movement is building self-esteem, there's no doubt that moving more can be helpful in burning off more energy, and, of course, that's going to help. If you're not the type of person who already loves running or spinning or cycling or CrossFit, that's not a problem. But it doesn't mean there aren't types of movement you've never tried that will make you feel alive. Be on the lookout for new types of movement practices and try to maintain the playful curiosity that kids naturally have when they're seeking new and innovative ways to move. Here are a few options you may not have considered.

Movement options to experiment with at home
All of the following movements can be done without going to a gym and without getting changed into "workout clothes." Choose a few that you like and do as much as you can.

- **Skipping**—fun and easy to do and makes you feel like a kid

- **Dancing**—it is almost impossible to dance to a positive, upbeat tune and not feel good about yourself

- **Jumping-jack intervals**—try doing them for thirty seconds and then resting for thirty seconds. Repeat as many times as you want

- **Sprinting in the backyard**

- **Five-minute yoga sequences**

Movement options to experiment with outside the home

Of course, it may also be worth considering a weekly class that you can attend that makes you feel good about yourself and more confident. This has the added benefit of connecting you with other like-minded people.

- **Nordic walking**

- **Indoor climbing**

- **Cycling groups**

- **Martial arts** (e.g. t'ai chi or qi gong)

- **Pilates**

- **Yoga**

- **Boxing**

- **Open-water swimming**—a super-fun way to challenge yourself and immerse yourself in nature

- **Salsa classes or ballroom dancing**

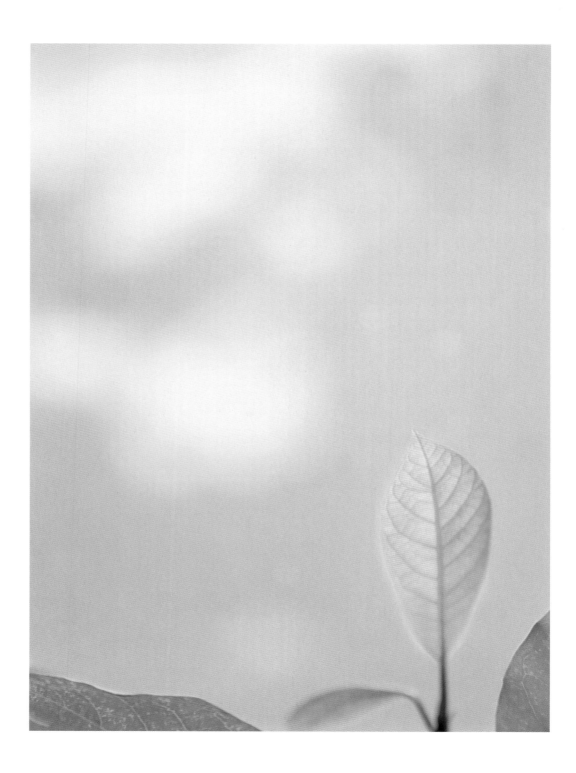

3

WHEN
WE
EAT

WHEN DO YOU EAT YOUR FOOD?

One of the most astonishing discoveries weight-loss researchers have made in recent years is that *when* we eat might be just as important as *what* we eat. Over the past few years, numerous studies have suggested that if you eat the majority of your calories earlier in the day, you can end up losing more weight than if you eat those same calories later on and into the evening.

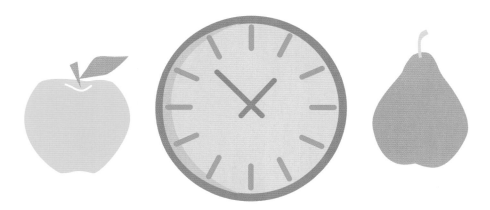

How could this possibly be? According to the old calories in/calories out theory, food is simply fuel. You put calories into your body, then your body burns up whatever it needs and stores the rest as fat. It shouldn't matter *when* you put the gas in your tank, or how often you fill up; all that matters is that there is fuel to burn. But what scientists now know is that the times of the day we choose to eat, and how often, can have a significant effect on how much weight we put on. This is because the timing and frequency of our food affects the working of our signals.

When thinking about *when* you eat, I want you to think about the following three questions:

1
How often do you snack during the day?

2
Do you eat the majority of your food in the first half of the day or the second half?

3
What time do you eat your first bite of food and what time do you eat your last?

A SNACK ATTACK

If you're trying to lose excess weight, it's a good idea to try to limit the number of times per day you're putting food into your mouth. This means cutting right back on snacking. One reason obesity has been soaring over the last few decades is that we've dramatically increased how frequently we're putting fuel into our systems. Back in the 1970s, most of us ate just three times per day—breakfast, lunch, and dinner. But things are very different now. One huge study that was carried out in the early 2000s found that people were, on average, eating six times per day. More recently, in 2015, a group of scientists gave people smartphone apps to record how often they ate. Only 10 percent were eating three times a day, as we were back in the 1970s. The top 10 percent were eating a whopping ten times a day! You don't need me to tell you that the more often you eat, the more likely it is that you will put on weight.

Our store-fat signals are influenced by the hormone insulin. Whenever we eat, insulin is released that informs our body that fuel has become available. It instructs the body not to break down the fat it already has onboard. So if you're eating small meals and snacks multiple times a day (especially if they are highly processed), your body is being flooded with regular releases of insulin, which means it is never being allowed to break its own energy stores down and is constantly stuck in the store-fat mode. Essentially, you are never giving your body enough of a break from food to allow it to start burning off your existing fat stores.

On top of this, it's becoming clear that regular eating can make us more hungry. The body gets used to regular top-ups, so begins demanding them. However, as I have seen with countless patients, once you get used to snacking less, your hunger levels respond and you stop feeling as hungry in between meals.

LIMIT SNACKING

Reduce the number of times you eat each day

I would encourage you to try and reduce how much you snack. There is nothing inherently wrong with snacking but, in my experience, there are two main reasons why you may be snacking more than you need to:

- You've not eaten enough at the previous meal. If you don't eat enough food at mealtimes, of course, you may end up with an irresistible urge to snack after a few hours. This can easily be fixed by eating more food at the preceding meal and/or experimenting with increasing your protein intake, which helps keep you full for longer.

- It's a habit you've picked up over time that may have more to do with boredom, stress, or loneliness. The tools in "Why We Eat" and, in particular, the Freedom Exercise on page 93 can help you tackle this.

If you do need to snack, I would recommend you choose wholefood options such as carrots and hummus, celery and nut butter, or a piece of fruit.

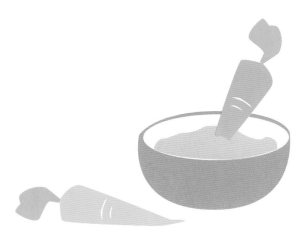

BREAKFAST LIKE A KING, LUNCH LIKE A PRINCE, DINE LIKE A PAUPER

This is one of those old-school sayings that has been passed down from generation to generation. But is there any truth to it? Well, as it turns out, there is. Eating most of our food earlier in the day rather than later seems to be better for our waistlines and our overall health.

Our body runs on daily rhythms and we process food differently at different times of the day. One weight-loss study put people on a diet where they would eat most of their calories in the first half of the day. Compared to the other group, who ate most of their calories in the second half of the day, the first group lost significantly more weight, even though the total amount of calories they ate was the same!

This adds to a growing body of research suggesting that any excess calories we consume at night are more likely to be stored as fat than those we consume in the morning. It seems we are simply not designed to be taking in and digesting food late into the evening.

When we eat earlier in the day, there tends to be a domino effect as to how many calories we consume afterwards. It positively affects our signals and, in particular, our hunger levels. I have seen over and over again with some of my patients that when they eat the bulk of their calories in the morning and early afternoon, they are less tempted to overeat and snack in the evening.

In contrast, many people who are trying to lose weight often end up "restricting" how much they eat in the daytime. They feel good about themselves during the day, but by the time they get home in the evening they are ravenous and often end up overeating to compensate.

CASE STUDY

This is exactly what happened to one of my patients, Alan. He was a forty-eight-year-old GP who had been trying to lose weight for years but never seemed to do it. He told me that he managed to be "good" throughout the day but it would all go pear-shaped in the evening. He was getting more and more frustrated. No matter what he tried, he just couldn't resist that evening blow-out. He would have what he considered to be a healthy smoothie in the morning, full of nuts, apples, and berries. At lunchtime, he would have a quick soup or egg salad from a local café. He was so busy throughout the day at work that he didn't really have much time to think about food, but when he would finally get home at 7:30 p.m., he'd be ravenous. He would happily tuck into his dinner, eat seconds, have a bit of dessert and often end up snacking on chips in front of the TV with a bottle of beer. The next day, the cycle would repeat again.

I suggested that he change his eating patterns and try to eat more for breakfast and less for dinner. It changed everything. Initially, it was a bit tougher, as he had to get up earlier and prepare his breakfast. He started the day with a two-egg omelette and some avocado or broccoli. At lunchtime, he would nip to the staff room and heat up leftovers from the night before. By early afternoon, he had eaten significantly more food than he was eating before. Remarkably, when he got home in the evening, he didn't feel that hungry. Dinnertime was typically where he got to catch up with his wife and kids, so he would sit with them and have a small salad or some soup. After a few days, he noticed his sleep had improved and his heartburn symptoms had gone. Over the next few months, he lost a significant amount of weight. Remarkably, it felt fairly effortless—all he had to do was eat most of his food earlier in the day.

Some people genuinely do not feel hungry first thing in the morning and don't want their first meal until mid-morning, or even later. This is completely fine—we are all different and it's certainly true that some people appear to thrive with this kind of eating pattern. However, the only reason that some of us don't feel peckish first thing is because we've eaten too late the night before. Many of my patients find they are breakfast people, but only once they change to an earlier evening meal time. Don't just assume you are not a breakfast person. Experiment and make sure!

MOVEMENT BEFORE BREAKFAST

Whenever you end up breaking your fast, you can score a massive weight-loss win by having a walk or a quick workout before you eat. Doing some form of physical activity, whether it be a twenty-minute walk or a five-minute body-weight strength workout, while your system is still relatively empty of fuel, will give you an extra dose of fat-burning right at the start of the day and help you keep your blood sugar under control.

EAT EARLIER IN THE DAY

Eat most of your calories before 3 p.m.

I'd like you to experiment with eating the majority of your food in the first half of the day—eating most of your calories before 3 p.m. works as a good guide for most.

Because of modern lifestyles and work patterns, I do recognize that eating earlier in the day can prove challenging. Like everything in this book, you do not need to adopt an all-or-nothing mindset. Small changes make a big difference. Perhaps you could shift your evening meal thirty minutes earlier? Or, maybe, you could experiment with lighter dinners and pay attention to the domino effects to your sleep quality, mood, and energy levels.

Or, maybe, this approach just won't work for you. That is completely okay. There are many ways to lose weight sustainably and the truth is that not all of my suggestions will work for you in the context of your life. You may find that restricting your eating window, as discussed shortly on pages 175–79, is a more realistic approach.

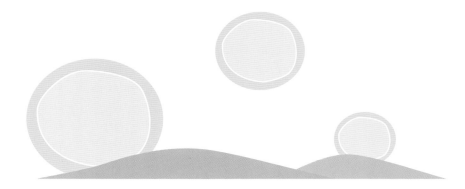

FOOD HANGOVERS

Have you ever woken up with a food hangover? You feel awful: fuzzy, headachey, dry-mouthed, fatigued, and like you've swallowed a greasy football. It's easy to assume this is caused by simply eating too much food the night before. But food hangovers aren't this straightforward. The hours you've spent asleep should, in theory, be plenty of time to allow you to digest even a super-large meal. Food hangovers aren't always caused by eating too much, but by eating too late.

If you eat a meal when your body isn't geared up to receive it, it's going to struggle. It's a little like being in an office, where different things are scheduled to happen at different times. The cleaners come in at 7 p.m. to vacuum and polish and empty the trash cans. If they came at noon, when you are in the middle of a presentation, there'd be chaos. The same thing is true of your digestive system. Around three hours before bedtime, the sleep hormone melatonin should start to flood your system, making you feel tired. The same hormone tells some of your organs to begin shutting down for rest, including ones that affect how you process food and store it as fat. This is why I'd like you to get into the habit of eating nothing for two, or preferably three, hours before bedtime. If you want to get to a healthy weight, it's much better to work with your body and not against it.

If you do work late, I would recommend that you try and eat your evening meal earlier, perhaps on one of your breaks. One of my patients regularly works shifts from 1 p.m. to 10 p.m. In the past, she would get home and eat around 10.30 p.m., but I encouraged her to take her dinner in with her and eat it during her 5.30 p.m. break. It was hard at first but, within days, she would find herself less hungry later on. She ended up sleeping better and found it much easier to make healthy food choices the following day.

"HUMANS DIDN'T EVOLVE TO HAVE FOOD CONSTANTLY IN THEIR SYSTEMS. WE'RE NOT DESIGNED TO BE DIGESTING FOOD ALL DAY LONG."

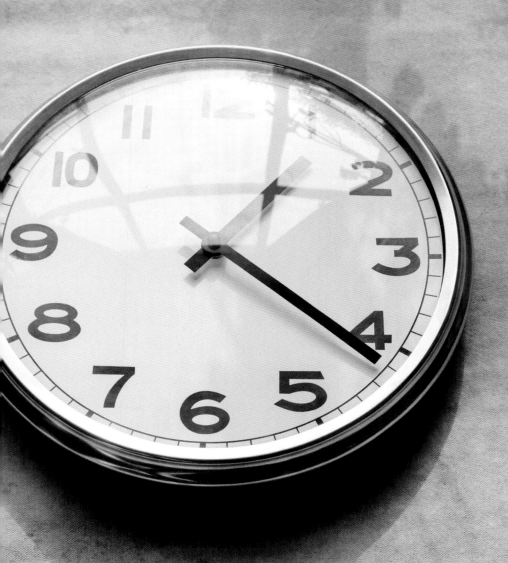

TIME-RESTRICTED EATING

Humans didn't evolve to have food constantly in their systems. We're not designed to be digesting food all day long. This is why reducing the hours in which we eat to a limited window can be a great idea. In 2018, one set of scientists compared a group of people who ate their meals over an entire day with those who ate all their meals within just eight hours. Remarkably, at the end of eight weeks, the second group, who did all their eating inside a compressed time window, showed a marked reduction in fat, even though the amount of calories eaten was the same between each group. Rather than changing *what* they ate, they changed *when* they ate.

Time-restricted eating has proved to be an effective strategy with plenty of my patients, readers, and podcast listeners. Many prefer to start off with a twelve-hour window (for example, eating between 8 a.m. and 8 p.m.), which should be manageable for most, and end up moving it down to ten or eight hours. My clinical experience has shown that, in isolation, it may not work for everyone when it comes to losing weight, but I would strongly encourage you to at least go for the twelve-hour window. Let's not forget, this was probably the norm for everyone on Earth as recently as fifty years ago. It's only because our eating habits have changed so much that we've had to give a special name to what's been a normal part of the human routine for ever.

HOW DOES TIME-RESTRICTED EATING WORK?

If you go online, you'll see hundreds of experts debating the merits of time-restricted eating. It's a hot new topic and there remains some disagreement, but this is how I see it: if you limit when you can eat, you're probably going to automatically reduce the number of calories you consume. This is obviously going to be helpful for losing excess weight.

But it's likely that time-restricted eating works in other ways, too, as it helps you work with your body's daily cycles, not against them. The latest science suggests that time-restricted eating reduces the body's store-fat signals and may even help you go the other way, turning your body into a fat-burning machine. When you haven't eaten for a few hours, your body starts to use up the fuel it's kept stored in places around your body, like your liver. This means storage space is created for the next time you eat. Once you start getting close to around twelve hours without taking in any food, your body's fat-burning will have increased significantly.

However, within about fifteen minutes of you taking in your first calorie of the day, you stop burning fat stores and focus on burning what you've just eaten instead. This is why having at least twelve hours without food in every twenty-four is so important. And, hopefully, you will be in bed for about eight of them!

Professor Satchin Panda, one of the world's leading experts in circadian biology, has shown that over 50 percent of adults eat their food over fifteen hours each day. And yes, this includes milk in your morning coffee or a glass of wine on the sofa at night! Therefore, these adults have only nine hours in each day when they are not taking in food—the only time they're

You can listen to more on the benefits of time-restricted eating in my conversation with Professor Panda on my *Feel Better, Live More* podcast at drchatterjee.com/81

not eating is when they're asleep! This is simply not enough time for them (or you!) to kick into full fat-burning mode.

An additional benefit of time-restricted eating is that it is highly effective at tackling hunger, once you get used to it. When you reduce your eating window, after a week or so your hunger signals outside that feeding window tend to go down.

I love time-restricted eating because it's brilliantly simple and fits around people's lives. It works with everyone's dietary preferences and it also allows flexibility. If, one evening, you're invited to a work night out and finish eating at 10 p.m., you can simply get back to your normal schedule the following day. Or, you can shift the next day's window further on and start eating at 10 a.m. and finish eating at your normal time. No problem.

If you've not tried it before, you should bear in mind that some people find the first week challenging. Please don't let this put you off. Your body just needs some adjustment time to get used to your new rhythm. If you are really struggling with hunger during that first week, some of the strategies on page 210 may help.

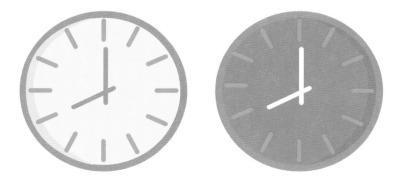

In addition to fat loss, restricting your eating window may also help you:

- Reduce hunger and snacking

- Improve sleep

- Improve digestive symptoms, like heartburn

- Stabilize blood sugar

- Support your immune system

- Increase energy

- Reduce inflammation

- Improve IBS symptoms

NB. Time-restricted eating is slightly different from the previous recommendation of trying to eat the majority of your food earlier in the day, although, of course, there can be an overlap. For example, you could choose an early eating window such as 8 a.m.–6 p.m., which will also result in you eating most of your food earlier in the day. However, there is not always an overlap and even later restricted-eating windows can be helpful. For example, one of my patients simply can't make an early breakfast work for him in the context of his lifestyle. He has found that a ten-hour eating window of 10 a.m.–8 p.m. works best for him—he can manage it regularly, it helps him sleep better, gives him more energy—and, of course, it helps him lose weight. Experiment and see what works best for you.

TAKE CONTROL OF YOUR EATING WINDOW

Try to eat all of your meals in under a twelve-hour window

Use the following tips to help you:

- Carefully document when you eat your first bite of food and when you eat your last bite over the course of a week

- Pick a twelve-hour window that fits your lifestyle, for example, start breakfast at 7 a.m. and finish dinner by 7 p.m. Don't feel disheartened if the first week is tough. Give your body time to adjust. Don't be afraid to try different eating windows to see if they work better

- Encourage any other adults in your household to participate. Behavior change is always easier when other people are involved, and it helps keep you motivated and accountable

- Pay attention to how you feel when you are eating this way. Does your hunger change? Do you sleep better? Do your symptoms of poor digestion improve? Write down any benefits daily. This is so useful, as it helps to really solidify those benefits in your mind

- When twelve hours becomes a breeze, experiment with eleven, and then ten. But don't push it too far beyond your comfort zone. What you're looking for is a way of eating that's sustainable in the long term

- Don't worry if you slip from time to time. It doesn't matter if you can't manage it every single day

- You can drink water, herbal teas, and non-sugared black tea or coffee outside your eating window

NB. If you have type 2 diabetes or are on any blood sugar lowering medications, talk to your doctor before you go for prolonged periods without eating.

CASE STUDY

I love it when small health interventions cause amazing, positive ripple effects. One of the most satisfying cases I've had recently was that of Shilpa. She'd been visibly overweight since childhood. Because her brothers, sister, and parents also had problems with their weight, she assumed it was in her genes and that there was nothing she could do about it. She worked as a PA at a prestigious law firm and I could tell that she was a naturally organized person who thrived on order, so I asked if she'd heard of time-restricted eating.

It turned out she hadn't. But she immediately liked the sound of it. We chatted about her eating schedule. She had a one-hour commute and would eat two slices of toast at around 6.30 a.m. before leaving for the station. She'd then get home at around 7.30 p.m. and would then eat dinner at 8 p.m. Finally, she'd curl up in front of the TV with a packet of sweets, which would usually last her until 10 p.m. This made her eating window just over fifteen hours.

Initially, I asked her to reduce it to twelve. Rather than having that toast in the morning, she would take a couple of boiled eggs into work with her and eat them around 8.30 a.m. She also tried to drop those after-dinner sweets, which she found really challenging at first. However, within days, she felt better. Her sleep quality had improved and she felt lighter and more energetic. She thought that she already slept pretty well, but when she woke up feeling ready to bounce out of bed, she realized how wrong she'd been. On her own, she moved her eating window down to ten hours, delaying breakfast until her mid-morning break at work. Over the course of a few weeks, she noticed that her IBS-type digestive symptoms had improved significantly as well.

Once Shilpa's body got used to her eating window, her system adapted and her signals changed so she felt less hungry. She was more productive at work and felt better about herself. She was also losing weight. In her enthusiasm, she decided to experiment with an eight-hour window but, finding she couldn't stick to it consistently, moved back to ten. Finding herself much more energetic in the evenings, she joined a martial arts class and attended twice a week, which was something she'd wanted to do all her life but had always felt she was too heavy. She took the lessons not to burn calories but because they made her feel good. But guess what? Her weight fell off. Within three months, she was slimmer than she'd ever been in her adult life, and she hadn't made many changes to her diet at all.

CHEATS, TREATS, AND FEASTS

Some popular diet programs talk about concepts like "cheat days" and "sinful" foods. While I understand the rationale behind this kind of language, I worry it can send out the wrong message about food. For me, it attaches too much moral judgement to our choices, and that risks putting us on a slippery slope to guilt, shame, and binge eating. But that said, for some people, knowing they have one day a week when they can just let it all blow out seems to work. I don't have a strict view on this. As with so many so-called rules about weight loss, there's no one-size-fits-all solution. If it works for you and helps you sustain a healthy weight, then go for it.

Other people might find it more helpful to make treats and feasts exactly that—rare occasions that are indulged in only occasionally, and with planning and purpose. This was brought home to me in a memorable incident a couple of years ago, when I was invited to Guernsey to give a lecture. During my stay, I was lucky enough to meet the island's oldest resident, a 102-year-old gentleman. When I got to his house I pressed the bell and waited. I'm used to doing home visits as a GP and, when I get to the door, the patient is usually too frail to let me in, so a carer or family member will assist, or we'll get access via a key that's been put in a safelock in the porch. But, to my astonishment, this extremely elderly man answered the door and greeted me with a big smile and an impressive handshake.

When I asked him about his favorite food, he beamed and told me all about a local delicacy called gâche, an amazing-sounding fruit bread made with raisins, sultanas, and cherries. "How often do you have it?" I asked. "Is it the kind of thing you have with tea each day, or only on Sundays?" He looked shocked at the thought. "I only eat it at Easter and at Christmas!" he said. This man was enjoying his blissy food, and he was loving it, but he was saving it for when there was something to genuinely celebrate, on scheduled feast days. Not only that, he didn't feel he was depriving himself the rest of the time.

I think we can all learn something from this wise centenarian's relationship with food. He consumed a sweet delicacy, that he loved, a mere two times a year. Yet, we now live in a society that encourages us to consume these kinds of blissy foods daily.

What are your favorite food delicacies? Is it a cream bun? Or, perhaps, you prefer a bag of chips? How often do you consume these foods? And, what do they really symbolize to you? These are the types of questions you will have to ask yourself if you are truly going to reset your relationship with food and lose weight for good.

One of my patients, Sally, a busy 46-year-old working mother with three children, told me that she has either a large bag of chips or a bar of chocolate four to five times per week in front of the television. After reflecting on the reasons why, she told me with absolute clarity that for her, eating the chips or chocolate bar symbolized "me-time." It was a sign to her that her kids were fast asleep in bed and her work for the day was done—the dishes were washed, her kitchen was clean, and all work emails had been sent. This was unadulterated time for herself— blissful time that she celebrated with blissy foods.

Once she understood what role this behavior served in her life, she was empowered to change her habits. She decided that instead of mindlessly consuming blissy food in front of the TV each evening, she would light a scented candle and sit there relaxing either reading or listen to music. The candle became her symbol of "me-time" rather than chips and chocolate. Over the coming weeks and months, she significantly reduced how often she would snack in the evenings and, in turn, her sleep quality improved and her weight started to come down.

Once you start to understand the role these foods play in your life, you too will become empowered to make changes.

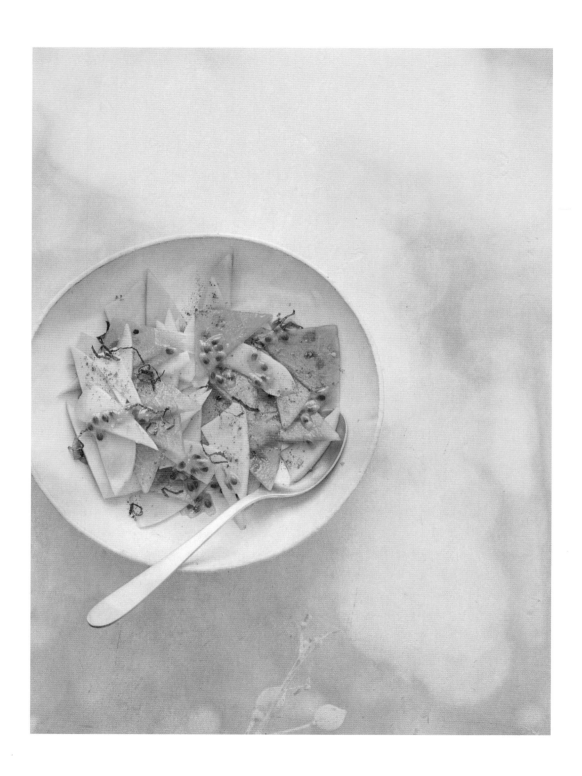

4

HOW WE EAT

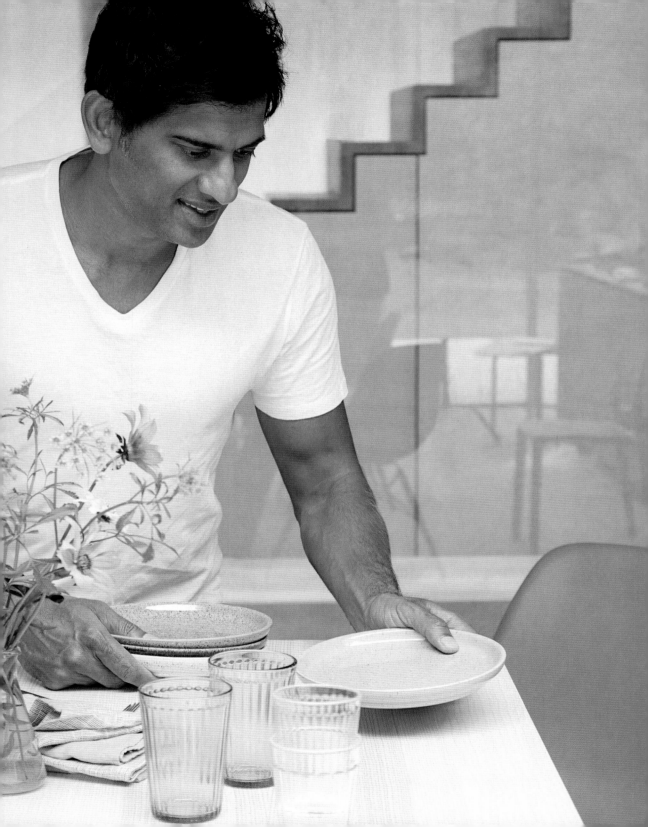

NOTICE
EVERY BITE

Our journey so far has told us that what we eat is crucial for dropping excess weight, and so is why we eat and when we eat. Now it's time to take a look at how we eat. Are we sitting down for meals with our loved ones, or are we eating alone? Are we having lunch al fresco or al desko? Are we eating mindfully and listening to our signals? Or are we distracted?

THE MYSTERY OF THE FRENCH

There's long been a mystery that's puzzled weight-loss scientists. It's sometimes known as "the French paradox." The mystery is this: why is it that, compared to the US, the French seem to be able to eat cheese and pastries and creamy sauces, all washed down with a glass of red wine, and still remain relatively slim?

There are a number of theories, but my view is that it is mostly to do with *how* they eat, rather than just *what* they eat. The French tend to eat when their bodies are in the optimal relaxed state to process food. Every lunchtime they lower their laptop lids, leave their desks or put down tools on whatever work they might be doing, and sit in the cafeteria or in a nearby café and eat lunch. By doing this they're putting their systems in a rest-and-digest state. They're focusing on enjoying the food on their plate and perhaps making easy conversation with friends, just as humans have been doing for tens of thousands of years. They might have a slice of cheese after lunch, but only a slice. They're not inhaling it mindlessly while they stare at a screen. And it is real cheese, not the highly processed, spreadable gunk that comes in a plastic tub and looks like toothpaste.

Contrast this with the average lunch break in the US. Sandwiches, chips, and a drink at your desk, reading emails, surfing social media, or catching up with the work that didn't get done in the morning. Over here, we have a desk-lunch culture and a work-late culture. It's the same in many countries around the world.

But why should this make a difference to our waistlines? Well, by now you will be more than familiar with the idea that if you want to lose weight successfully and then keep it off, it's best to get your body's signals working properly. If you don't, you'll be fighting hunger and triggering your body to store fat in ways that won't be helpful. But once you have your signals working properly, it's important to make sure you can actually hear them. If you're eating while you're distracted, and thinking about a million other things, it's going to be much harder to hear the signal that's telling you you've had enough.

Scientific research shows this to be true. One study found that "being distracted or not paying attention to a meal" tended to make people eat more. But if they did pay attention to what they were eating, not only would they eat less at that sitting, they'd eat less later on that day. In other words, if you eat in front of the television, you'll eat more. If you eat in front of your computer, you'll eat more. If you eat while scrolling down your phone, you'll eat more. But if you make time for your food, and don't treat it as a chore that you have to deal with while multitasking the rest of your life, you'll feel satisfied with less, for longer.

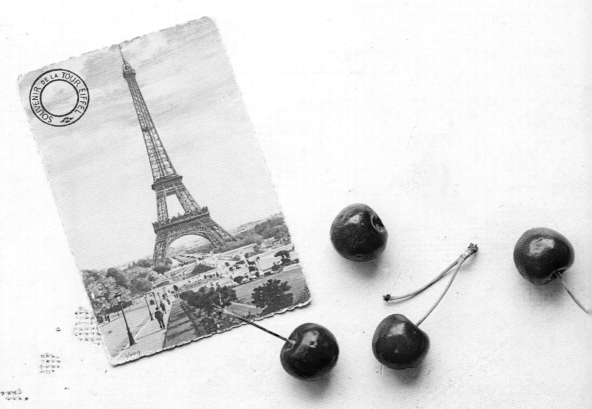

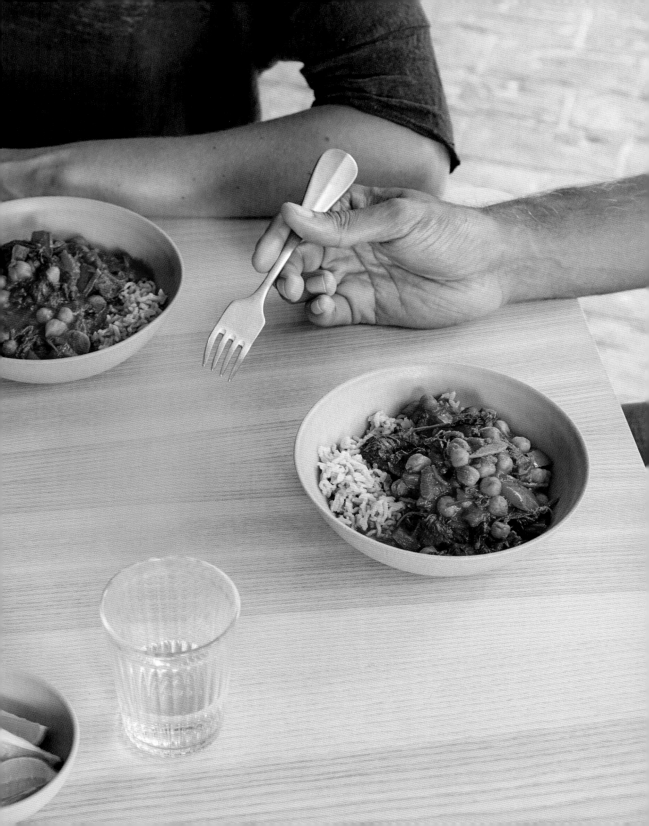

EATING TOGETHER

It's easy to underestimate the importance of eating in company. It was only when I was filming a BBC TV series, *Doctor in the House*, and I went and lived alongside families that I realized that so many of us are not eating together at all. On my very first night with a family I was startled to see them all having their evening meal separately. Dad was eating standing up in the kitchen, Mom was on one edge of an L-shaped sofa watching TV, the teenage daughter was on the other end of the sofa on Facebook, and the teenage son was sitting at the table doing emails. As I continued filming up and down the country, I saw this scene repeated over and over again.

None of them were really paying attention to what they were eating. Having a meal was just something to do while they got on with something else that seemed more important. And it's not just about distraction. Scientists have found that the act of eating together helps us bond and feel connected. According to one famous psychologist, Professor Robin Dunbar, this can have "profound effects on our physical and mental health, our happiness and wellbeing, and even our sense of purpose in life." But surveys show that we're eating alone more and more. One found that, over the course of a week, almost 50 percent of meals in the UK were eaten alone, and that 34 percent of Britons can go an entire week without eating in the company of anyone else. I agree with Professor Dunbar, who says that, "joining in communal meals is perhaps the single most important thing we can do—both for our own health and wellbeing and for that of the wider community."

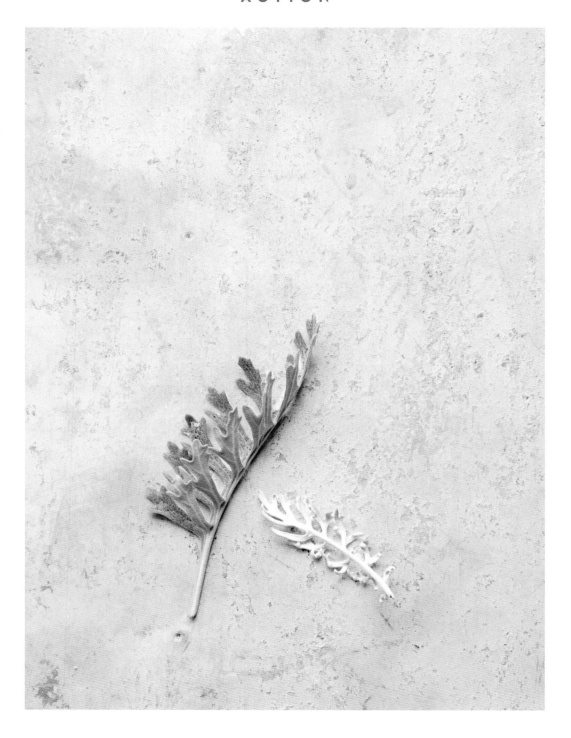

EAT WITH OTHERS, NOT WITH DEVICES

Eat at a table with others (no TV or phone!)

Try to eat as many meals as you can with other people. It could be with your family, partner, or roommate at home and, maybe, a colleague at work. If possible, turn your phone off (or leave in another room) and eat at a table away from your computer or television.

Sitting at a table helps connect you to the people you are with and encourages you to put the brakes on whatever else is going on in your life—it signals to your body that it is time to switch off and eat.

Of course, not everyone has loved ones or friends they can regularly eat with. If you live alone, while it is tempting to give yourself "company" with your smartphone or television, I would really encourage you to try and eat without them. You can achieve wonderful benefits by sitting in silence and really paying attention to your meal. Take your time and, if you can, mindfully chew each mouthful ten to twenty times. You'll experience different tastes and sensations and be more satisfied with less.

If you really struggle to eat in silence, as many people do, why not try having some relaxing music on in the background instead of the television. It's more likely that you will eat more mindfully and less likely that you will overeat. As with everything in this book, experiment and see what works best for you.

TEN MINUTES OF SOLITUDE

Take 10 minutes each day to focus on yourself

Just as important as eating in company is taking time for yourself alone, to really tune in to how you're feeling. Building awareness of your body's signals means getting into the habit of spending time in peace, every day, and really listening to them. I'd love you to spend ten minutes each day in silence, without your smartphone and without the world sucking up and stealing your attention. Switch off your computer, turn off social media and turn your attention inwards. This is time for you to rest your body and nourish your mind.

Here are a few ideas to get you started:

- Meditation—try an app like Calm or Headspace if you have never done this before

- A practice of mindfulness like a crossword or an adult coloring book

- Listening to relaxing music (without looking at your phone!)

- A cup of coffee in complete silence with no music, smartphones, or distraction

- A breathing practice, like the one on page 123.
  Or, visit drchatterjee.com/breathing to see some different techniques

- Journaling—try writing down any thoughts or worries in a journal each day. This can help us feel calmer and less anxious

In my experience, this tends to work best for most people first thing in the morning, often as part of a morning routine. Other fixed times in your day which you might want to stick this practice on to are with a morning cup of tea, on your commute to work, at lunchtime, or in the evening before bed. Pick a time that works for you and your lifestyle.

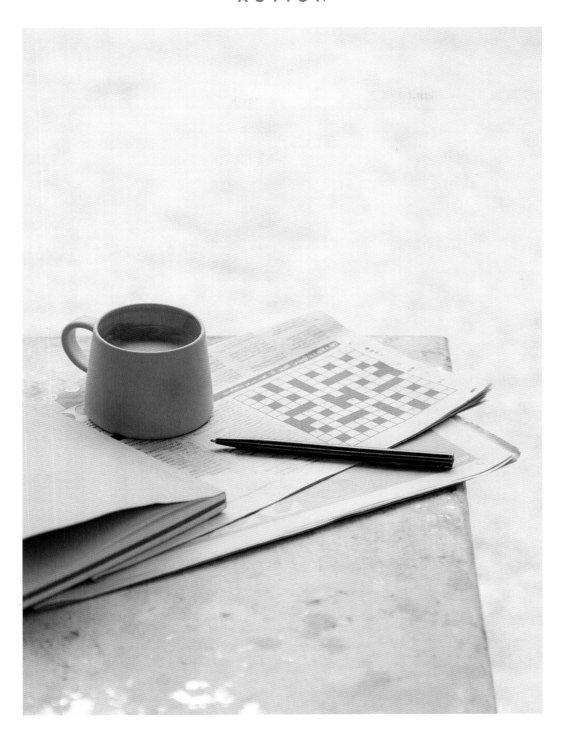

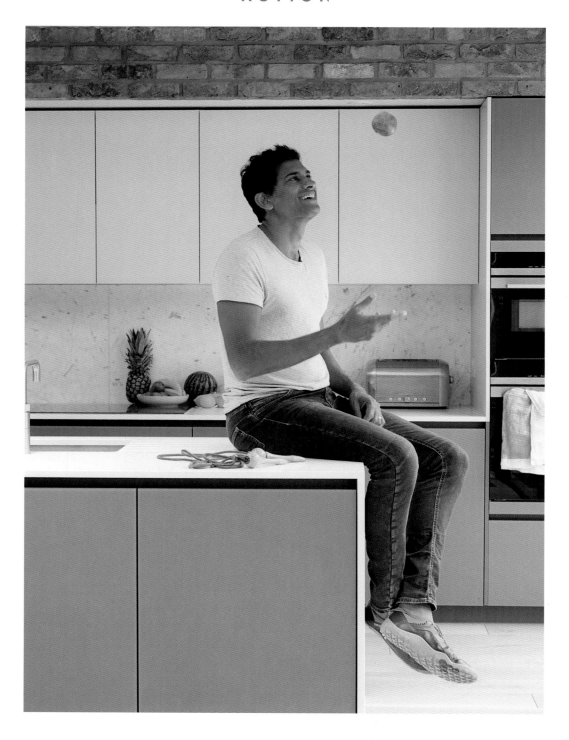

MAKE COOKING TIME FUN

Make cooking a special time for you

There's no getting away from it: cooking the same meals day in, day out, can feel like a chore. But I think it's possible to reframe cooking. In my house, I've turned it into a fun, chilled-out time when I can properly relax and enjoy my own company. It just took the introduction of some simple rules. I put my laptop away and leave my phone in another room so I can't be distracted by emails and calls, and I try and make sure the kids are engaged in a fun activity in another room. Then I put some of my favorite music on my kitchen CD player and have a blast. Sure, I might be making a fool of myself as I sing along and play the odd bit of air guitar on a silicon spatula, but nobody can see me (and who cares if they do!) and it's great for my sense of joy and wellbeing. While I'm cooking I also try and tidy up and get the table ready. When I'm done, there's a lovely sense of satisfaction and achievement from preparing something tasty and nourishing for my family.

HARA HACHI BU

The Japanese are a bit like the French in that, for various cultural reasons, they suffer far less from obesity than many developed nations. For example, they have a cultural practice called hara hachi bu, which means that you eat until you're 80 percent full. Of course, nobody's measuring when they're exactly 80 percent full. The idea is to be mindful of how full you're getting and eat at a measured pace. You can judge for yourself when you're 80 percent full, then get into the habit of leaving what's left.

We're simply not used to thinking about our differing levels of fullness in the West. Often we're only really aware of two states—starving and stuffed. We've got stretch receptors on our stomach so, when we start to eat, and the stomach begins to expand, it starts to send the fullness signal out. Feeling uncomfortably bloated is a sign that we've gone past full and our body is in distress. It's a sign that something's gone wrong, like a pain signal, but we often take it to be a good thing.

Some of us are even guilty of instilling this idea in our kids. We have a habit of telling them, "You've got to eat everything on your plate," or even "You can't have dessert until you've finished your main." I suspect this comes from our parents and grandparents and is a hangover from a time when food was scarce. It was an appropriate response to that environment, but it's not any more. In fact, today's problem is the opposite. We're surrounded by an abundance of cheap, energy-dense food. We're rewarding children for going past full and their prize is often a fatty, sugary dessert. This eat-up mindset is no longer fit for purpose. I'd argue that it's time we made our children feel good when they choose not to eat to bursting, rather than when they do.

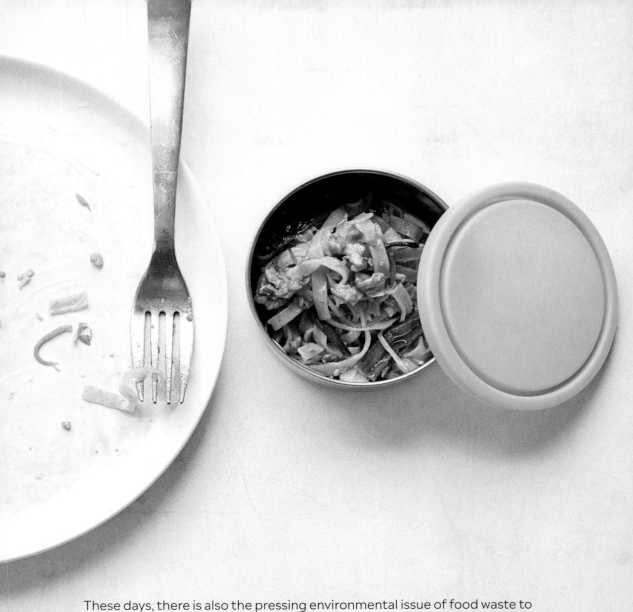

These days, there is also the pressing environmental issue of food waste to consider, so I would encourage you to not pile your plate up too high in the first place. Also, try and keep all leftovers to use up the next day for a quick and healthy lunch in the office, or, perhaps, in your children's lunchbox.

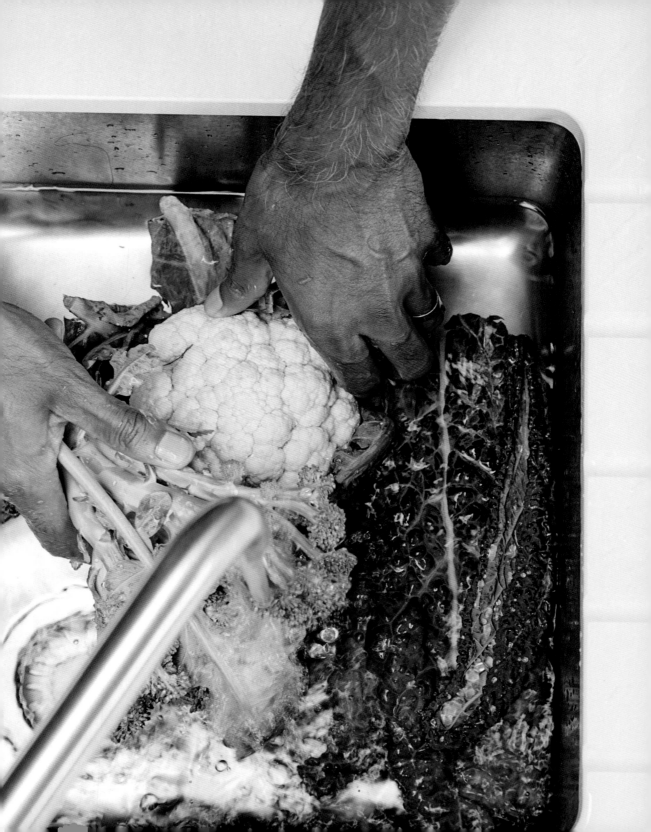

THE CHEWABILITY FACTOR

A huge part of being a mindful eater is not eating too quickly. Choosing the right kinds of foods to eat can be a huge help with this. Imagine you have six apples on a plate in front of you. You're told to eat them. You'll probably feel full long before you get to apple number six. This is partly because the apple has fiber in it, which makes it harder to chew. Now imagine that someone has juiced those same six apples into a small glass and told you to drink it. That's going down your throat in a couple of gulps. It's the same food, containing the same amount of sugar, but you consumed it in seconds—and it doesn't even help you feel full.

This is why I'd like you to consider the chewability factor of the food you're eating. Slices of roast beef, a whole chicken breast, or a portion of steamed vegetables takes a bit of chewing, and this forces you to slow down. When you slow down, you'll experience the fullness signal properly and automatically become a more mindful eater. When I was at university, the local pizza restaurant had "all you can eat" buffets for $5 on Wednesday nights. My friends and I would go and stuff as much of it down our necks as we could. Back then, I was super-competitive and my trick was to eat as quickly as possible. I'd tell my friends, "You've got to get it in before your stomach realizes that you're full! You guys aren't eating quickly enough!"

And, I was right. The fullness signal takes time to trigger. Modern fast food like pizza and French fries has been designed to be practically inhaled. But you have to take your time over a roast dinner or a full breakfast, cutting pieces up and layering them on to a fork.

So real food takes longer to eat. But this isn't its only advantage. It's also typically richer in fiber, which has multiple benefits, such as slower absorption, which also means your blood sugar remains more stable. A brilliant trick I use to slow me down is to fill up half my plate with non-starchy veggies like broccoli, kale, cauliflower and Brussels sprouts, and make sure I eat them first. This way, I'm slowed down and filled up, the reverse of my younger self competitively eating pizza.

EAT MINDFULLY

When you are finally sat down in front of your food, there are several practices that you can adopt while eating that will help you slow down, pay attention to every bite, and notice your body's signals.

Eating mindfully means that you are paying attention to the fact that you are eating. It means that you are not being distracted by other activities and tasks but, instead, are focussed only on your meal. When we eat mindfully, we experience more flavor and taste from our food and will often end up eating less.

Experiment with some of the following tips and see what works well for you:

- Chew each mouthful 10–20 times and notice the enhanced flavors on your taste-buds

- Put your cutlery down between each mouthful

- Eat foods that require you to chew for longer. These are minimally processed foods that are close to their natural state. Examples include non-starchy vegetables (e.g., carrots, broccoli, cauliflower, lettuce), fresh fruit (e.g., apples and pears), meat, and fish

- Eat until you are 80% full, like the Japanese do

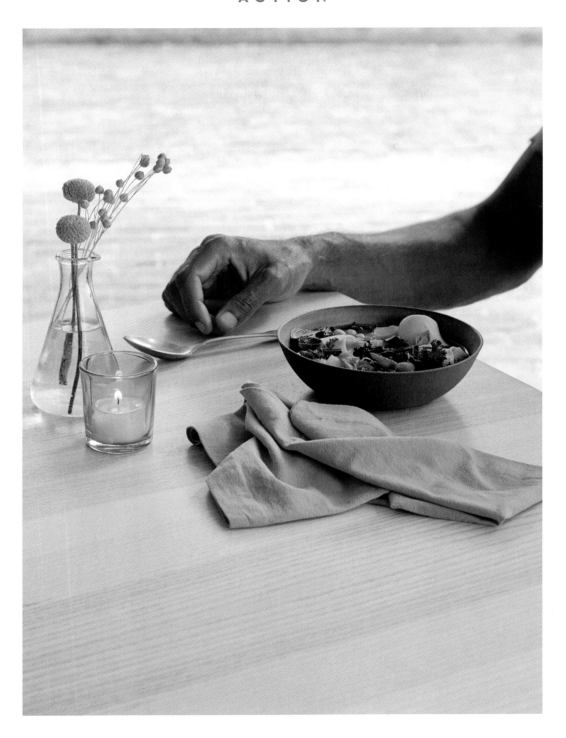

A MINDFUL MOMENT OF BLISS

Next time you have an overwhelming urge to eat something sweet and blissy, don't try and resist. Instead, eat the food you are itching to consume, but try to do so slowly and mindfully.

1

Sit down in a quiet room away from distractions.

2

Look at the piece of food and be aware of how you're feeling. Are you excited? Can you feel your stomach juices start to flow? Can you feel saliva being released into your mouth in anticipation?

3

Acknowledge any guilt and shame you may feel and try to put it to one side.

4

Focus on the experience of slowly unwrapping and/or feeling the texture. Spend a moment luxuriating in the smell.

5

Allow it to sit on your tongue for a few seconds. Notice how you become aware of different tastes you haven't noticed before.

6

Enjoy it, savor it, as slowly as possible. Focus on the taste and the texture.

Continually assess how you feel. Does one bite scratch your itch? Has your mood changed? Was the first bite the best? Did subsequent bites deliver diminishing returns? My patients often find that the first few bites were all that they needed. Or, sometimes, they realize that it wasn't actually food that they were craving. This exercise is well worth repeating regularly.

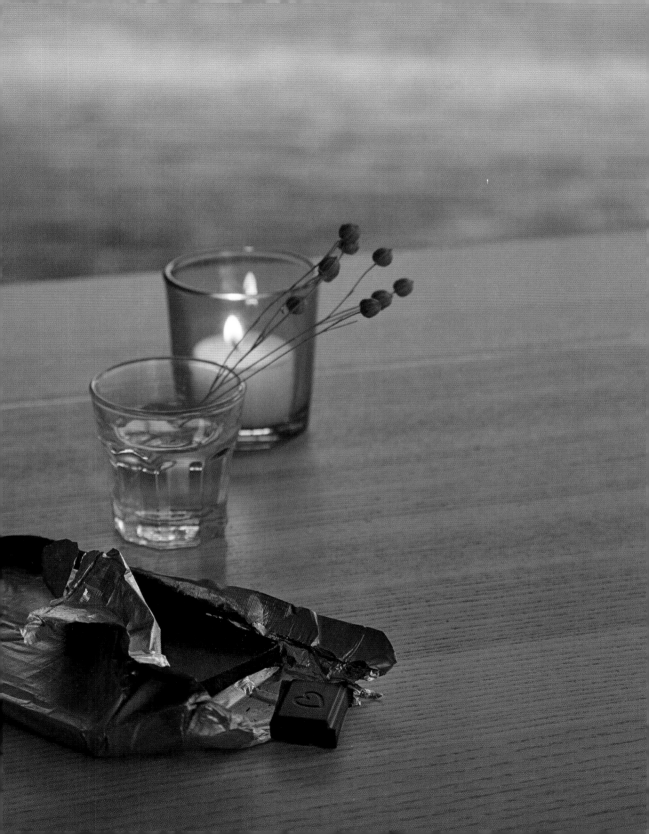

TRANSITION TIMES

It's just so easy to slip into mindless eating. Much of the time we're rushing around and when and if we do get round to putting food inside our mouths, before we know it, our plates are empty and we don't quite know how. That's if we even took the time to use a plate in the first place!

The good news is, it's easy to interrupt this habit by using simple transition times that help get you out of action mode and into rest-and-digest mode, which is your body's optimal state to receive and process food. This means your body will deal with food more efficiently, which means you're less likely to overeat. It also means you may end up storing less of it as fat.

I think of this as having a high performance strategy for eating. Just as an athlete seeks high performance in their sport by preparing their bodies and minds beforehand, I'd love you to seek high performance for mindful eating by using transition times to prepare yourself to process meals in an optimal way.

TELL YOUR BODY IT'S TIME TO EAT

Spend a few moments preparing your body for food

Before you start eating it's a good idea to help your body get into its optimal state for digesting food by taking a few moments to prepare.

Here are some options to help you design your own personalized strategy—experiment and choose the ones that work best for you.

- Turn off all electronic devices or put them in another room

- Do a few minutes of meditation

- Do one minute of breathwork—many patients love my 3–4–5 breathing technique just before meals (drchatterjee.com/3-4-5) or try the five-finger breathing routine on page 96

- Do one minute of exercise—jumping jacks, push-ups, and dancing are great options

- Go for a quick five-minute walk around the block

- Clean your kitchen table and light some candles

- Take your pulse for fifteen seconds. This helps you tune into your bodily sensations

- Try turning off any music. The fewer the distractions, the more likely you are to pay attention to what you are eating. If you do choose to have music in the background, make sure it is calm and relaxing

- Just before you eat, have ten seconds of gratitude (see page 209)

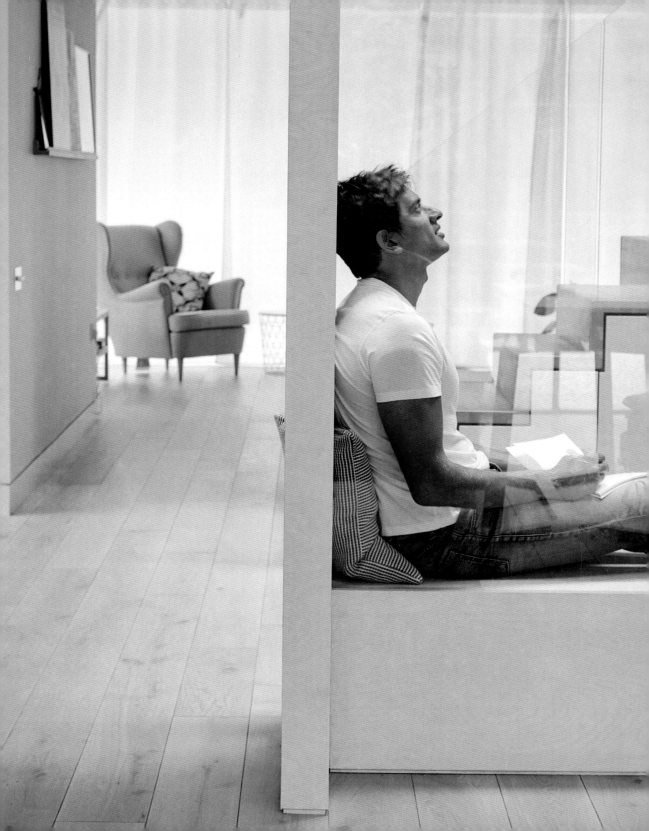

TEN SECONDS OF GRATITUDE

Lots of us are familiar with the old Christian practice of saying a prayer of thanks called grace before eating. Hindus do something similar. In fact, this is a norm in many cultures around the world and, no matter how religious you are, I believe it's one of those products of ancient wisdom that we could all learn something from. All you need to do is find a phrase that works for you.

Here are a few ideas, but please feel free to make up your own:

1

Thank you [name of person who cooked the meal] for making this delicious meal.

2

Thank you [name of person who provided the food] for giving us this meal.

3

Thank you all for taking time to enjoy this food together.

4

I am thankful for the food I am about to receive.

5

Hara hachi bu (the Okinawans, in Japan, say this phrase before every meal) or *I will eat until I am 80 percent full* (the English translation of hara hachi bu!).

6

Thank you to Mother Nature for providing this wonderful meal.

Taking ten seconds to pause before eating and marking your gratitude helps enormously with eating more mindfully. If you're eating with others, it really helps build that connection and emphasizes that the meal you're about to share is something you're doing together.

ZAP YOUR CRAVINGS

As you've already learned in this chapter, eating in company, eating more slowly, and having a pause before each meal helps you to eat more mindfully. This usually results in people eating less when they eat as they feel full earlier. It can also result in them experiencing fewer cravings afterwards. I have seen this with so many of my patients—that when they pay attention to how they eat, their cravings outside mealtimes plummet as well.

Some people, though, will still experience difficult cravings outside mealtimes and may need other strategies to help. Over time, taking a small pause and doing the Freedom Exercise on page 93 will help you understand the causes of your cravings, which often come from stress and emotions, rather than hunger.

In the meantime, you may need a short term fix for when those difficult cravings strike. In my experience, one of the most effective strategies to zap your cravings is to distract yourself by shifting your focus onto something else.

You could try:

- **Doing a quick workout**

- **Having a large drink of water**

- **Doing a short meditation or breathing exercise**

- **Popping to the bathroom**

- **Stealing a cuddle from one of your kids, partner, or a pet**

- **Moving to a different room**

If, despite these tactics, you are still struggling with a strong craving for something sweet, try having a piece of fruit.

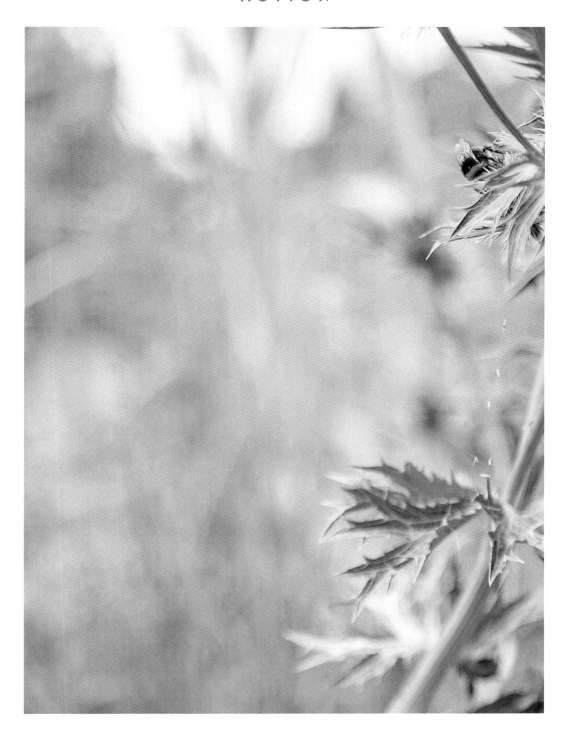

"EATING MINDFULLY HELPS YOU EAT LESS AND CRAVE LESS."

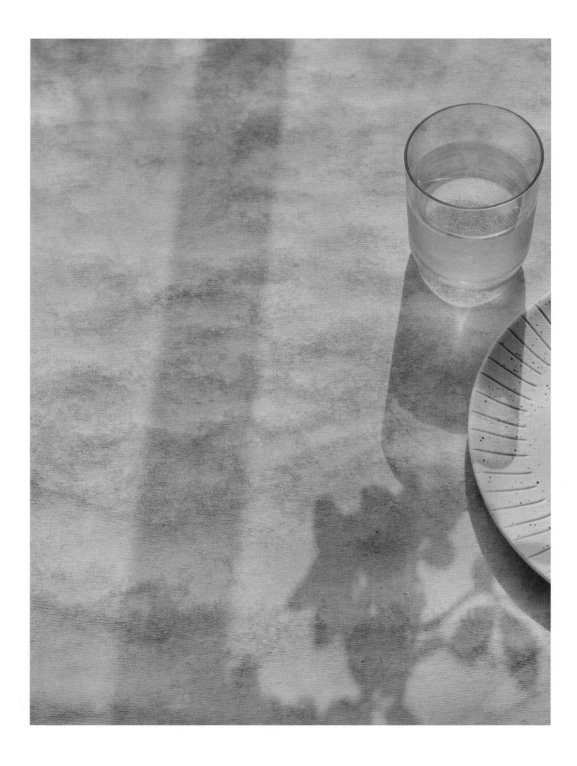

5

WHERE

WE

EAT

YOUR ENVIRONMENT MATTERS

(MORE THAN YOU THINK)

London's Euston Station must be one of the unhealthiest places in the country. It's a vast hall, seemingly always crammed with tired and stressed-out people, and its walls are lined with shops that sell sweets, fries, and sugary drinks, and with fast-food outlets that pump the tempting scents of cooking meat and bread out over the crowds. I spend a lot of time at Euston because it's where I catch my train back home up north. Time and time again I've found myself there, exhausted and irritable, staring at bags of tempting sweets. And, on many occasions, I'll crack. I'll look over my shoulder to check I've not been spotted, grab what I want, rush to the checkout, and then hide the bag in my coat pocket, shoving the sweets in my mouth one by one. But afterwards, when I'm on the train, I don't beat myself up like I used to. Yes, I cracked. But that doesn't mean I'm a bad person. It means I'm tired, stressed, tempted, and human.

In a way, all of modern life is a bit like Euston Station. You could hardly design a better scenario than normal life in the twenty-first century for making a lot of people overweight. As we've been finding out, we're a sleep-deprived people and that makes us crave more calorie-dense foods. Our jobs make us sit at desks and in trains, buses, and cars, so we're not moving enough to send our bodies the signal that we are active, thriving humans. We're stressed out in our work, family, and home lives, which makes our bodies think we're in a hostile place, so they hold on to more fat. On top of all that, it's hard for many of us to get easy access to healthy and affordable wholefoods.

And what's the result? Soaring obesity rates. In 1992, 53 percent of the UK population were overweight or obese. In just twenty years that number has climbed to 62 percent. And it's still climbing. Maybe your parents' and grandparents' generation could get away with eating whatever they wanted, but they weren't living in the world of today. They didn't have access to the types and varieties of foods that we do. At the start of this journey, I explained that it's not your fault if you're carrying excess weight. By now, I hope you agree.

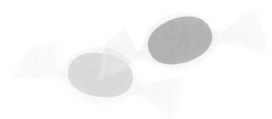

OUR ETERNAL SUMMER

People who live in areas of the world, like Okinawa in Japan, that don't have high rates of obesity and other health problems aren't trying to be healthy. They have no choice but to walk to see their friends. There are no offices for them to work in or desks for them to get stuck behind. The cheapest food on offer just happens to be the healthiest. They don't suffer chronic stress and they have a strong sense of community. They don't have more willpower than us, or more motivation. Their environment just happens to be set up in such a way that good health is the most likely outcome.

It's just not like this in most Western communities. We're surrounded by blissy foods, and that's enormously triggering for our brains. One study found that if there are more than six fast-food restaurants within half a mile of your house, you're 40 percent more likely to be obese than if there are three. Part of the reason for this is that we're wired to experience a spike of desire and craving for these foods even at the sight or smell of them. When you smell a cheeseburger or see the logo of your favorite fast-food brand, your brain begins its learned program of driving you to get some (page 34). The more of these types of foods we've eaten in our lives, the stronger this urge will be and the more likely our brain will succeed in its goal of finding it and eating it.

On top of this, we're wired to scarf down sweet, carby, calorie-dense foods whenever we see them, even if they are so-called "healthy" foods. For much of our past, we'd only encounter foods like berries, fruits, honey, grains, and

To hear more about the powerful effect of the environment on our behavior, listen to an incredible conversation I had with Dan Buettner on my *Feel Better, Live More* podcast at drchatterjee.com/67

root veggies in the summer or early autumn. We're designed to want to eat as much of it as we can in order to store fuel for the tough, lean winter. Some experts have pointed out that we're living in a kind of endless summer. We are preparing our bodies for winter, but winter never actually comes! For the first time in human history, we can get sweet foods 365 days a year, easily and cheaply. But the wiring in our brain doesn't know this. All it knows is, whenever it's surrounded by lovely sweetness, we're supposed to consume as much of it as we can.

Fighting all this means fighting millions of years of evolution. When we gorge on sweet things, our brains and bodies are doing exactly what they're supposed to do. We do have a certain amount of willpower to work against this programming but, needless to say, it's limited.

What's worse, many of us live in areas where it's really quite challenging to get hold of healthy food. I used to work in a GP practice in Oldham, Manchester, where I'd work with my patients, trying to empower them to eat well. One day I forgot my packed lunch and had to go out in search of something healthy to eat. It was close to impossible. I walked past at least ten fried-chicken and kebab shops before the option of anything healthy popped up, and they all had huge posters in the window advertising large meals for £1.99. The reality hit me so hard that day, I'll never forget it. I knew I could give the best advice in the world but the families I was treating would then walk out into a food landscape where the healthy choice would end up being the most difficult choice, as well as the most expensive one.

BUILD YOURSELF AN IGLOO
IN THE BLIZZARD OF FAT

I've got a friend who has a really problematic relationship with food. He and his wife fall out all the time because he just cannot resist a packet of cookies. His wife thinks he's being pathetic. "Why can't you just say no?" she says. "I can. It's easy. I just don't eat them." But, in all likelihood, she's wired differently to him. She experiences the sight and smell of that packet of cookies, and the desire for blissy food, in a different way to him. It's much easier for her to say no.

I think most of us would accept that, if we were living with an alcoholic, we probably wouldn't keep alcohol in the house. What we need to realize is that the same reward systems and compulsive behaviors are at play when someone has a problematic relationship with blissy food. While the situations aren't identical, they are comparable. It's craving, compulsion, temptation, willpower, and anxiety. I think we should take our problematic food habits just as seriously as we take problematic alcohol habits. If we're struggling with excess weight, that means making our homes free of unnecessary temptation. We're being set up to fail whenever we leave the house because of food adverts, tempting shop displays, appealing packaging, and the mouthwatering smell of delights such as freshly baked croissants. When you're out there, you have to use willpower all the time. If you have to use it inside your house, too, you're destined for failure.

I can be as bad as anyone. If I've got a packet of chips somewhere in the house, there's no way I won't eat them. The moment I feel tired and stressed, I'll be there, ripping it open. This is why, before you begin your weight-loss journey, I'd like you to make your home a safe shelter from the blizzard of temptation that exists outside it. Most of the decisions we make every day are a consequence of the environment we happen to be in. We're constantly being nudged and triggered into actions by the things that sur-round us. Research has suggested that people who have cereal boxes or toasters visible and easily accessible on their kitchen counter weigh more than those who don't. I'm sure not all of that extra weight is just coming from the cereal or the toast, but it is an indication of just how powerful envi-ronments are in shaping us. If we see a toaster every time we walk into the kitchen, we're far more likely to trigger the brain into beginning its eat-toast program—especially when we're tired and peckish.

It's a great idea to make it just a little bit more inconvenient to get hold of blissy foods. I have a patient, John, who found chips hard to resist. We discussed strategies to make this behavior harder. He wouldn't agree to completely keep them out of the house (yet!), but he was happy to put them in the garden shed in a plastic bag. It meant that on a cold, wet evening, often he simply could not bear the thought of venturing out to the shed to get any. His chip consumption plummeted.

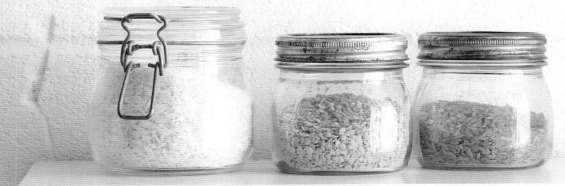

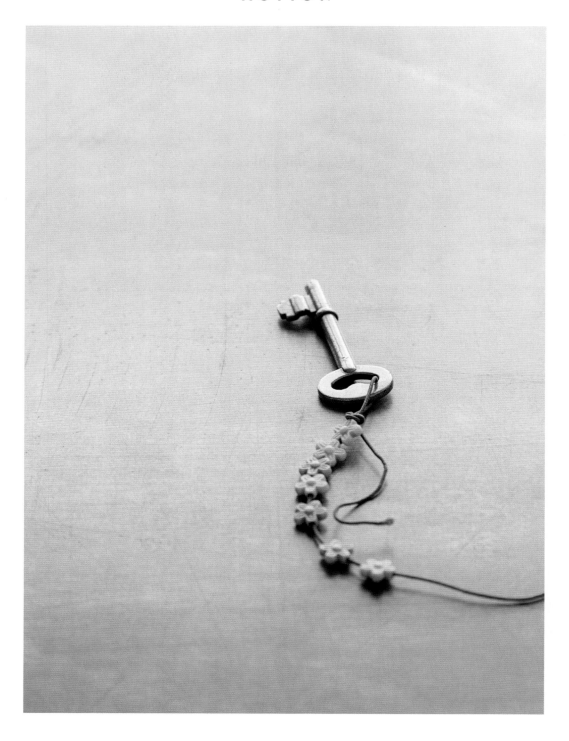

SIX WAYS TO RESIST TEMPTATION

Here are six strategies you can implement at home to make it harder to engage in behaviors you are actively trying to avoid or reduce.

1

Don't keep blissy foods such as ice cream, sweets, chocolates, and cookies in your house.

2

Don't bring juices or sodas home. Liquid energy is an unnecessary calorie bomb.

3

If your microwave is used regularly for highly processed ready meals, consider ditching it.

4

Once you've served dinner, put any leftovers in a container ready to go in the fridge before you start eating.

5

If you have a toast habit, get rid of your toaster or put it in a cupboard that you don't use often.

6

Keep any alcohol or blissy foods in your garden shed or loft, if you decide you don't want to get rid of them altogether. If you are trying to cut down on alcohol, try putting your wine bottle in the freezer either after you have poured yourself a glass or beforehand—it makes it just that little bit harder to pour yourself a second glass.

SIX WAYS TO SET UP YOUR HOME FOR SUCCESS

We can also tweak our home environment in simple ways that make it easier for us to engage in healthy behaviors. Here are six tips that you may wish to consider:

1

Keep a water bottle or jug visible. Make it attractive so you feel great when you see it. If helpful, put some chopped cucumber, sliced orange, or fresh mint in the water.

2

Keep vegetables at eye level in the fridge, not hidden in the bottom drawers.

3

Keep a kettlebell or dumb-bell in the kitchen by the kettle. Each time you walk by, you are being visually prompted to pick it up. Why not do some bicep curls every time you walk by? Before you know it, this will seem effortless and a normal everyday habit, just like brushing your teeth.

4

Ditch the scales. If our weight goes up by two pounds, we think we've done something bad. If it drops, we think we've done something good. In reality, we've often done nothing different. Weight can fluctuate by up to ten pounds a day. Some studies suggest using scales can even slow weight loss as they can encourage people to go off plan if they are not making the progress they think they should be making.

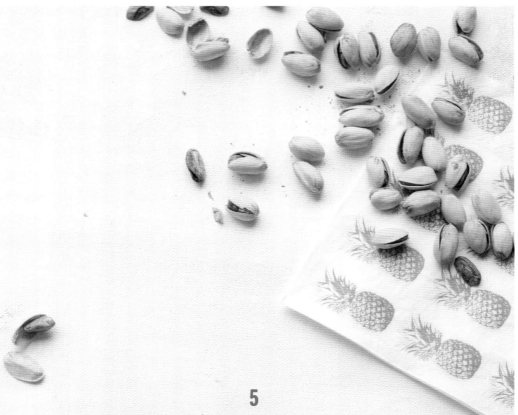

5

Keep your bedroom clean and calm. Have a dim bedside light by your bed, to encourage reading. Move your phone charger outside the bedroom. Consider removing your television. Keep a journal on your bedside table so that it is easy to do your daily reflection (see page 111) or to write down your worries or to-do list before you go to sleep.

6

Keep fruit and unsalted nuts, preferably still in their shells, in your home for times when you really need a snack. Removing the shell requires effort before you can eat them, which makes them harder to gorge on. Unsalted also makes it less likely you will overeat as the food is less "blissy."

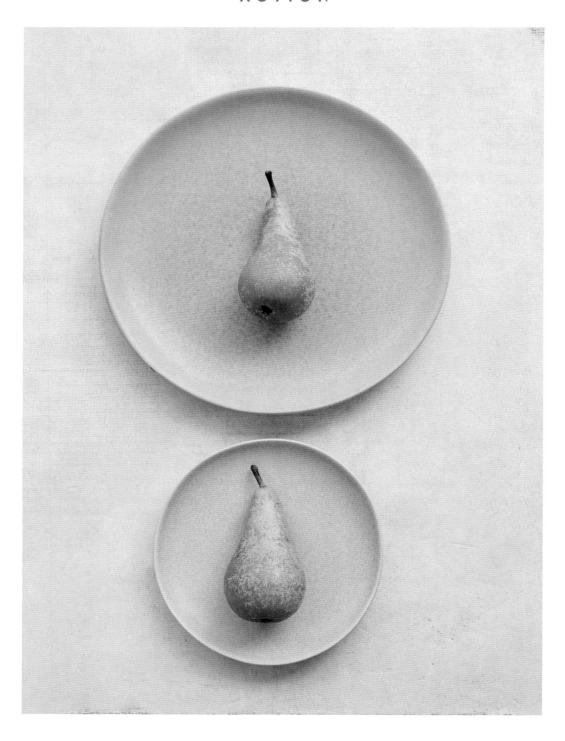

EAT OFF SMALLER PLATES

One handy hack that's great for tweaking your hunger signals is eating your meals off smaller plates. Surprisingly, there doesn't currently seem to be any reliable scientific research on this, but many of my patients have reported it works really well for them, and that's good enough evidence for me. They tell me that reducing the size of their plate by a couple of inches nudges them into eating smaller portions and being satisfied with less.

This is probably because, when we're judging anything like a portion size, the brain always does so by making a comparison. What's a large coffee in Starbucks? It's the one that's bigger than the medium. The same is true for food portions. One of the reasons some of us struggle to lose excess weight is because we are eating too much. A decent-sized meal will look plentiful on a smaller plate. But put it on a large one and it will seem small.

MAKE A MEAL PLAN

Plan ahead to avoid wasting food and making decisions out of hunger

Another way to keep your home environment working with you is to plan meals ahead. When you come home from work after a long day, motivation is often at its lowest, so it's hard to persuade yourself to take the time to cook something healthy. It can also be hard when you feel exhausted to actually decide what to cook. Patient after patient has told me that planning their meals in advance was a game-changer. It helps address decision-making fatigue (particularly at the end of the week!), and if you make a plan for the entire week and buy only what's needed, you also save quite a bit of money and avoid wasting food. Online shopping is best, if it's an option for you, as it removes the temptation to throw more than you need into the shopping cart.

Bonus tip: Always try your best to shop (online or instore) on a full stomach—we all know the perils of shopping when hungry!

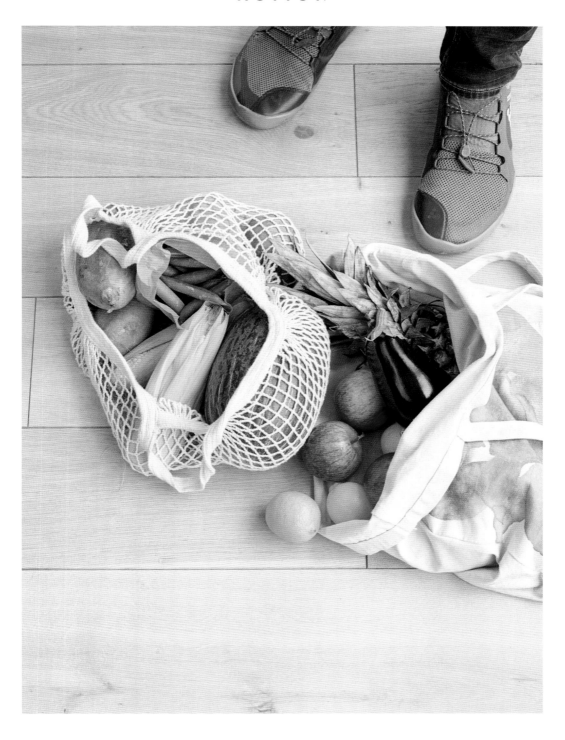

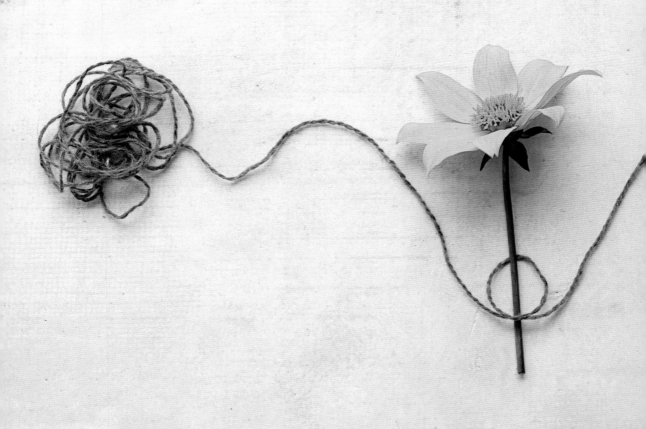

NETWORKS MATTER

Last Christmas, I went out for dinner with a couple of old schoolfriends. When it was time to look at the dessert menu, one of them said, mockingly, "Here we go, Rangan's going to do his healthy-eating thing again." I have to be honest, this made me feel slightly uncomfortable. I know he genuinely didn't mean anything by it, and to him it was only a small and harmless joke, but I felt a little excluded and judged. I also felt a lot of social pressure to join them in their sugary third course. When I got home and had the chance to reflect, I couldn't help but wonder what difference it made to him whether I ate dessert or not. Was the truth that he felt slightly guilty about his indulgence and that my not joining in made him feel worse? Were my choices acting as a mirror and reflecting back to him choices that he himself was not entirely happy with?

I can't possibly know. But I do know that our social networks can make a huge impact on how much excess weight we're carrying. Some truly extraordinary work by the researcher Nicholas Christakis has shone a light on how behaviors can flow through networks of thousands of people. He found that if someone in your immediate social circle becomes obese, you become around 45 percent more likely to be obese yourself. If a friend of one of your friends becomes obese, your chances of being affected increase by 25 percent. And, amazingly, if a friend of a friend of one of your friends becomes obese, your chances of being obese still climb by 10 percent.

This might be a hard thing to read and, of course, I'm not asking you to ditch your friends. But I do think you need to be mindful of the power of their presence in your life. If they put pressure on you to eat foods you're trying to avoid, could you sit down with them and let them know how much their support means to you? Could you explain to them that when they eat those foods in front of you it sabotages your efforts to improve your health? If that doesn't work, can you go for a few weeks without seeing them? Or, perhaps you could persuade them to join you on your weight-loss journey?

Similarly, we've already learned that stress can be a significant driver of weight gain. If people you follow on social media frequently post things that make you angry or upset, ask yourself if they're helping you. If not, I'd encourage you to mute or unfollow them.

The good news is that all this works the other way too. If you have healthy people in your life, you're much more likely to be healthier yourself.

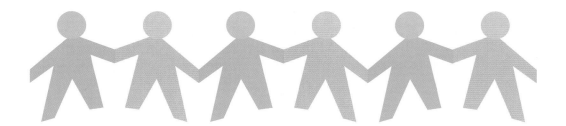

FIND A TRIBE OF COMRADES

I'd like you to make sure you have access to people that will support you on your weight-loss journey. Having access to your own tribe that is trying to engage in the same behaviors as you is extremely powerful. Here are some ideas that may help:

- Add some new friends into your life, who already engage in the behaviors that you desire. Do you have friends or work colleagues who are active, prioritize healthy eating, and help support the people around them? Perhaps, you could ask them if they would be up for a meet up or dinner once a week. Or, maybe, you could set up a dedicated WhatsApp group together to provide ongoing support, understanding, and motivation. If you already have friends like these, make an effort to see them or communicate with them regularly.

- Join a local class or group that will help connect you to like-minded people in your neighborhood. Examples might be yoga, pilates, martial arts, or dancing. Pick something that you've always wanted to do and something that will make you feel good. Of course, a lot of activities can be done and learned through the internet these days, but there is something powerful about connecting in person with people who have similar interests.

- Join a supportive online community. Many of my patients find gathering a network of comrades around them online can be a huge help. If you are struggling to find one, I'd love to see you on my own Facebook community (facebook.com/groups/drchatterjeetribe/) which is full of like-minded people who are supporting each other on their health journeys. We'd all love to see you on there!

CASE STUDY

Sheila was a busy working mom of three. By the time she got home from the office, she'd have just about enough energy left to "stay motivated" to cook a healthy meal for the children. Her husband would get back from work just after 8 p.m. and she'd watch TV with him. They used to love snacking together in front of some easy reality TV—it was their bonding time and a precious part of the day. When she was feeling especially bad about her weight, she'd try to say no to the chips or chocolate cookies, but having them right there in front of her was too much of a temptation.

When I asked if she could clean all the blissy food out of her home, she said she couldn't. Her kids liked to snack, and so did her husband—it wouldn't be fair to do that to them. So I asked Sheila if she felt those foods were helping her loved ones with their own health. She shook her head. Had she ever told them how she felt? She shook her head again.

I advised that one day soon, when she wasn't feeling angry or upset, she should explain how she felt to her family. She chose a Sunday morning after a chilled family breakfast. She announced she had something important to say and explained that she really wanted to look after herself. She was tired of being tired; she really wanted to improve the way she felt about herself and lose weight. She told them how important it was to her and asked them to help her. She understood that they wanted those foods in the house but said that it was almost impossible for her to resist them.

When she'd finished, her kids put their arms around her waist. Her husband said of course he would help: he only brought the cookies and chips into the house because he thought that's what she wanted. They agreed that once every two weeks they'd go out at the weekend as a family and have whatever they wanted. She removed the foods she was trying to avoid from her cupboards and dropped them off at a local food bank.

Now, whenever Sheila craved a snack in the evenings, all she would find in her cupboards were olives and nuts. She'd initially feel frustrated but then realize she wasn't really hungry at all. She was just bored. She and her husband soon realized the only reason they were up late watching TV was as an excuse to eat blissy foods. They started turning the TV off earlier and going to bed sooner. This triggered a classic ripple effect, as Sheila woke up with more energy and motivation. She began preparing a wholefood breakfast for the family every morning, which meant that she and her husband only needed a light lunch to keep them going until the evening. She started going to a salsa class twice a week. Two years later, she's absolutely thriving.

OUTSIDE OF THE HOME

From nearly two decades spent working within the UK's National Health Service, I know that our work environments can be places of near-constant temptation. The open tub of chocolates is a regular sight in doctors' receptions and hospital wards. It's a sad fact that 57 percent of NHS employees are either overweight or obese. These are amazing people who've devoted their lives to looking after others and keeping others healthy, and yet their work environments are making it challenging for them to look after themselves.

It's the same in many workplaces around the country. Employees who wish to make healthy choices are constantly having to fight their environment. And, as we've learned, the environment usually wins.

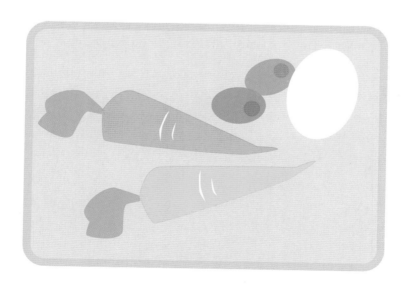

If this feels like something you need help with, I recommend you take some positive steps to defend yourself. Here are six tips that you might find useful:

- **Bringing your own food to work.**

- **Devoting some of your time off to food prep:** put on some relaxing tunes and cook some of your favorite meals in large batches that you can store in the fridge and take into work each day.

- **Enjoying a filling first meal of the day before you come into work.** If you're a breakfast person, have one rich in protein, such as eggs, salmon, or tofu. This helps keep you full and will reduce your desire to snack and your cravings.

- **Bringing a water bottle into work with you.** Try and drink the whole bottle before lunch, fill up at lunchtime, and finish the second bottle before you leave in the afternoon. When we drink enough water, we often crave snacks less.

- **Keeping an emergency snack pack with you for those times when you get really hungry and there's nothing healthy around.** Nuts, olives, carrots and hummus, eggs, cans of wild salmon, seeds, or leftovers are all great options.

- **Talking to work colleagues who like bringing in sweets and cakes.** Calmly, and in a nonjudgmental manner, explain that you find it hard to resist those foods and that you're trying really hard to look after yourself.

WHY SCHOOLS NEED A FOOD REVOLUTION

As a parent of two young kids, another environment that concerns me is schools. Recently, my wife and I looked around a series of high schools. We were surprised to see that all of them had vending machines in the corridors, selling sweets, chips, chocolates, and sodas. Lots also had cafeterias that sold the same things. One school even had an ice-cream van that visited its grounds every lunchtime. When I asked a principal about this, he said that they wanted to give their pupils "choice." This is a common response, but it demonstrates a huge lack of understanding, not only about how the brain works but also about how brilliant junk-food companies are at manipulating it. Most psychologists will tell you we have far less free will than we think. We're controlled largely by our subconscious minds, and they can be nudged and trained, not least by food corporations who tweak their food and marketing to make it much more likely we'll "choose" their products over others.

This wouldn't be such a big deal if obesity wasn't such a huge and pressing issue. But it's the biggest health crisis in the world, killing far more people than even the worst modern pandemic. One fifth of elementary school-children and a third of those at high school are overweight or obese.

I believe schools should be a model for our young people educationally, behaviorally, and nutritionally. Children and young adults learn a sense of what is acceptable in the world at school. They also learn what social norms are. Making highly processed, high-sugar foods so readily available sends a strong subconscious message to them that it is normal to have these foods around all the time and consume them at will. By doing this, we are unintentionally colluding with junk-food corporations. We are undermining all the parents who are desperate to raise their children to be aware of the real dangers of blissy foods. What's more, if these youngsters are able to resist the sweets and "treats," they risk becoming social outcasts at school.

Research has shown that if teachers make it a rule that pupils can't eat in corridors or in classrooms, the school's obesity rate lowers by 11 percent. When pupils eat real wholefood, their energy goes up, their school performance goes up, their cognition goes up, and their mental health improves.

A food revolution will benefit the schools themselves as much as their pupils. What teacher wouldn't want students who are more alert, more able to concentrate, and with better overall mental health? It's time to stand up and demand something better. Our kids deserve it.

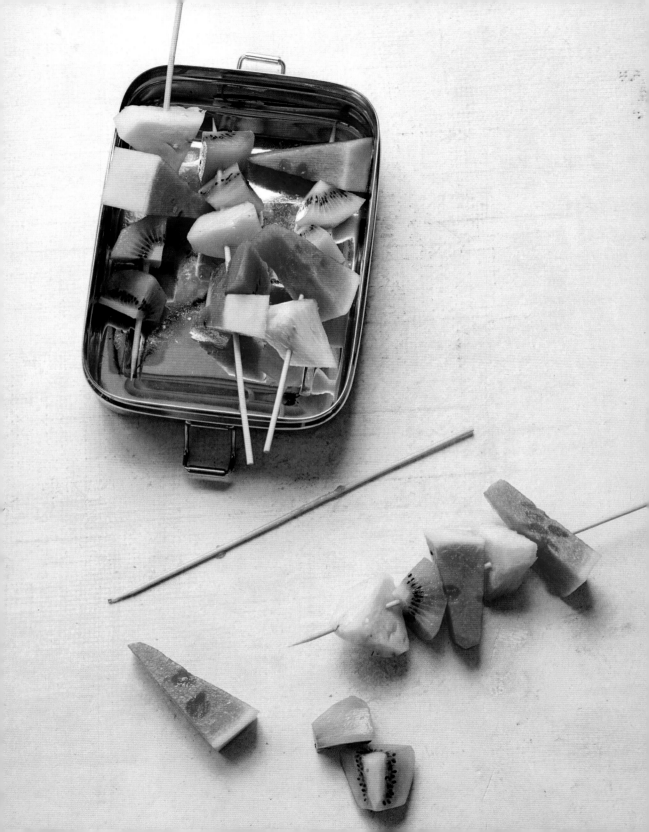

WHAT CAN YOU DO RIGHT NOW

While we wait for the school environment to change, here are some practical, positive steps you can take right now:

- **Send your child into school with some healthy snacks** like fruit, olives, or chopped-up crunchy veggies such as carrots and cucumber.

- **Try and ensure they have a nourishing breakfast,** rich in protein, before they leave for school. This will keep them fuller for longer and encourage less snacking. It will also help improve their focus and concentration.

- **Try not to bring chocolates or sweets into school premises when picking up your kids**. I completely respect your right to feed your children however you want, but remember this can make it harder for the families around you who are trying to make different choices.

- **For school trips or other special occasions, try packing them fruit kebabs.** We did this when my son was at his first elementary school: all the kids kept asking him about them and the teachers thought they were great and decided that they were going to suggest this for all future school trips. Often, people around you want to change but don't know how to. This is a great way of helping your own kids and inspiring change around them.

STAND UP FOR CHANGE

As well as adopting the strategies above about how to defend yourself from unhelpful environments outside the home, I would urge you to advocate for change in our schools and workplaces. If the environments outside our homes made the healthy choice the easy choice, instantaneously, millions of us would be healthier and happier without even trying. And it is not just the health of the individuals that would benefit. Employers would benefit from increased performance and less absenteeism, and schools would have happier and more engaged students.

If you feel as strongly about this as I do and want to get involved, please visit my website, where I have a guide to writing to those in power, whether it be the school principal or your employer, to remove vending machines, offer healthy options and remove any temptation that will test your willpower to the brink. On there you'll find two sample letters I've written for you to use. Feel free to tweak and modify them as you see fit.

If you want to send a letter to your employer advocating for workplace change, visit drchatterjee.com/workplace.

If, like me, you are a concerned parent, and you'd like to get involved with a food revolution in schools, please go to drchatterjee.com/schools.

In fact, why not put this book down and do it right now! You can print off the letters and post them, or simply send them by email. Encourage your friends and colleagues to do the same and, once you've done it, take a photo and post it on social media with the #schoolrevolution or #workplacerevolution.

Together, I'm convinced we can make a change.

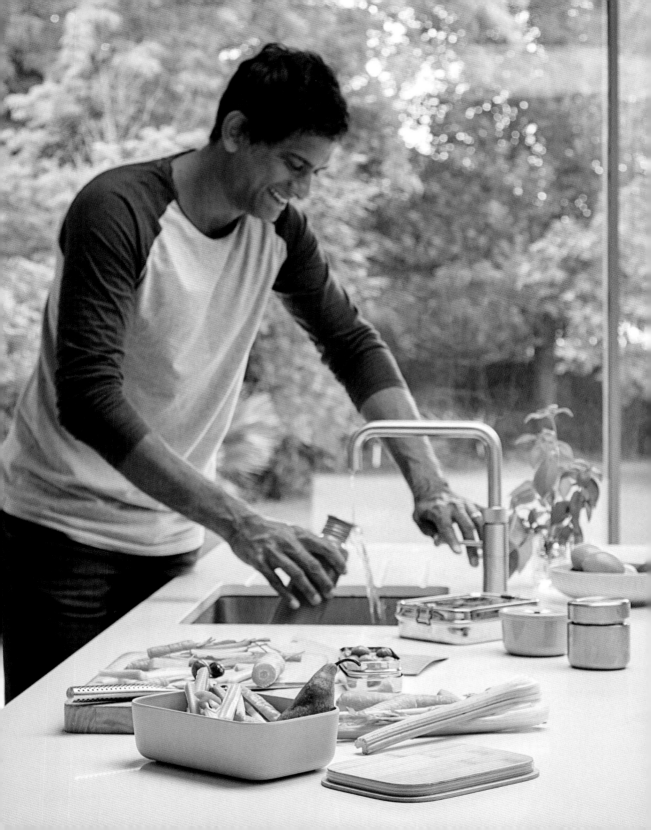

HOW TO DO

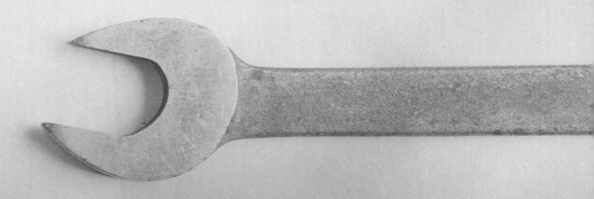

By now, I hope you have a much better understanding of the wide variety of factors that might be at play in determining your weight. As we've been discovering, there are so many different things that can contribute to weight gain that it's just not possible to design a one-size-fits-all weight-loss plan.

You are, of course, free to implement the tips in this book in any way you choose, but if you prefer a bit more structure, as many people do, I have

YOUR PLAN

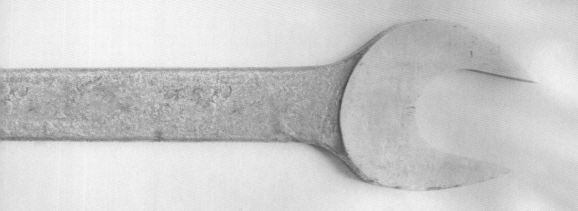

created some guidance for you. It's based upon what I have seen work successfully time and time again with my patients over the past 20 years.

I want you to become your own mechanic. I want to help you understand how unique your body and life history are and enable you to create your own bespoke plan. You're the expert in your own life, not me. I can give you the tools but, to truly succeed, you need to be in charge.

PREPARATION

While the temptation may be to jump straight in, it is essential to first spend a week or so getting ready for the journey on which you're about to embark. Put aside some time to really understand how to best tailor the plan to maximize your chances of long term success.

What's the most important factor for you to address first? Is it your self-esteem? Is it a lack of movement? Is it that you don't prioritize your sleep and therefore are trying to lose weight with one hand tied behind your back? Or, is it the way you have set up your home environment? Your road map to success will be unique to you.

I'd like you to think about the preparation phase as comprising of two different parts: preparation of your mind and preparation of your environment.

PREPARE YOUR MIND

Getting your mind right for the journey ahead is a crucial component of any weight-loss plan. Sit down in a quiet space with a pen and paper and answer the following questions.

- **Why do I want to lose weight?** List the benefits.

- **How much of my diet consists of "real food"?**

- **Do I sleep enough to feel refreshed?** If not, why not?

- **When stressed, what do I use to soothe my emotions?** It may be food, alcohol, social media, or something else entirely.

- **What movement do I do on a daily basis?** How much do I walk? What movements would I like to bring into my life?

- **Do I eat mindfully?** Or do I eat while in a rush and distracted?

- **How frequently do I eat every day?** What time do I start, and what time do I finish?

- **What do I think is my main obstacle or obstacles to losing weight?**

When you've finished, write down a positive statement about what you consider your top priorities to be. Examples include:

- **I want to improve the quality of my sleep.**

- **I want to see if I can use something other than food to soothe my emotions.**

- **When I feel bored, I will phone a friend or a relative, instead of turning to food.**

- **I will only bring foods into my house that nourish my body and mind.**

These positive statements will help you decide which actions you are going to focus on, when you design your very own plan on page 258. It is well worth revisiting this exercise every few weeks to reassess and see if any of your priorities have changed.

PREPARE YOUR ENVIRONMENT

Your environment exerts a powerful influence on the choices you make. I would strongly recommend that you control the environments that you can control. Spend some time this week preparing them as best you can.

- **Prepare your food environment**—Your home and, if possible, work environments should be stripped of temptations and filled with healthy nudges. This is one of the most powerful and effective things you can do. (See pages 223, 224, and 237.)

- **Prepare your sleep environment**—Make it easier to fall into a deep, relaxing sleep by removing temptations from your bedroom, such as televisions, laptops, and tablets. I would encourage you to charge your smartphone outside your bedroom and if you need an alarm, simply pick one up from a thrift shop or online. Make sure your curtains are effectively blocking out light or think about getting some blackout blinds. Eye masks, ear plugs, and blue light-blocking glasses can also be helpful.

- **Prepare your friends, family, and tribes**—Humans are social animals. If we want to succeed, the support of our networks can be crucial. Tell your friends, family, and work colleagues what your plans are and that you would like their support. (See pages 231–35.)

- **Prepare your shopping**—Write a meal plan for the week and plan to do your shop at a time when you are not tired, hungry, or stressed. Shopping online can be a great way to reduce temptation and you can set it up so that the nourishing foods you are trying to eat regularly automatically go on your list. Shopping well leads to eating well. Plan your shop carefully. (See page 228.)

NOW YOU'VE PREPARED, IT'S TIME TO START

THE TOOLBOX

Over the next few pages, I will introduce you to the *Feel Great, Lose Weight* toolbox. Within it, you have everything you need to lose weight for good. It comprises of:

3 x FOUNDATIONS

3 x EVERYDAY HABITS

3 x BOOSTERS

Like all toolboxes, some tools are essential and foundational for all of us. Other tools, however, are dependent on our individual situation and the specific issue we are trying to address.

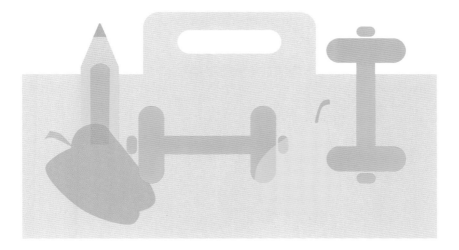

3 x FOUNDATIONS

These are the three core foundations of fat loss, which I want you, over time, to infuse in as much of your life as possible. Try your best to make small changes in each of them, to the best of your ability. Please remember that these foundations are areas that can always be improved. I have been focusing on them for years and I am still making small tweaks in them. That is part of the process.

Don't worry about getting them all perfect from day one. This is not a conventional "plan" where you have to have completed specific tasks in week 1, week 2, week 3, etc. before moving on. My approach is all about progress, not perfection. Please don't punish yourself if your progress isn't as quick as you'd like. Small changes made consistently over time is what leads to the big results.

It's possible that the "Prepare Your Mind" exercise on page 247 will have identified that one of these foundations requires more attention than the others. If this is the case, I would encourage you to focus on that foundation first. You will experience more benefits from small improvements in your weakest area, rather than making your strongest one even better.

In fact, many people are much more successful when they focus on only one foundation at any one time. When we try and change too much at once, it can quickly become overwhelming.

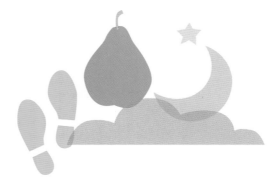

1 EAT REAL FOOD (AS MUCH AS YOU CAN)

Real food gets your signals working properly and helps you lose weight without making you feel too hungry. I want you to choose minimally processed food that's as close to its natural state as possible. Below are the tips that will help you do this. You do not need to follow all of them. Choose the ones that you think will work for you and your life.

- **Focus on One-Ingredient Foods** (page 45)
- **Dinner for Breakfast** (page 57)
- **Power Up With Protein** (page 58)
- **Greens Go First** (page 61)
- **Quench Your Hunger** (page 62)
- **Learn To Cook** (page 65)
- **Zap Your Cravings** (page 210)

2 MAKE SLEEP A PRIORITY

Not sleeping well makes you hungrier, makes you crave more sugary food, makes it easier for you to put on weight, makes you more emotional, and makes it harder for you to resist temptation. Getting sleep right makes everything else easier. For most of us, a few small lifestyle tweaks is all that is required. Use the tips below to help you. You do not need to follow all of them but the more of them you do, the more likely it is that the quality and length of your sleep will improve.

- **Get at least 20 minutes of natural light every morning.** (page 120)

- **Enjoy drinking caffeine in the morning—stop at noon.** (page 117)

- **Try and eat at least 2-3 hours before bed.** (page 172)

- **Try and minimize bright light exposure throughout the evenings.** (page 121)

- **Ensure the 1 hour before bed is as relaxing as possible—ideas for activities include yoga, stretching, breathing, journaling, and listening to music.** (page 121)

- **Bedtime Breathing Practice** (page 123)

- **Bedtime Journal** (page 118)

3 ALWAYS CHOOSE TO WALK

Choose every opportunity that you can to walk. Walking is the most fundamental human movement (see page 157). Simply walking as much as you can sends your body the signal that you're a thriving individual who's engaging with life. Use the tips below to help you.

(If you're unable to walk for any reason, use the suggestions on page 160–161 to find another form of movement you can enjoy.)

- **Consider walking to work, school, or the store**
- **Get off the bus a few stops early or park farther away**
- **Try a quick five-to-ten minute walk before breakfast or go up and down your stairs a few times**
- **Walk fifteen minutes every lunchtime (in nature if possible)**
- **Try a quick walk around the block before dinner and/or after dinner**
- **Try standing when using public transport**
- **Consider joining a local walking group**
- **Schedule regular walks with friends as a way of catching up**
- **Consider having walking meetings at work**

3 x EVERYDAY HABITS

The simplest and most effective way to start is by introducing these 3 daily habits into your life. They are easy to implement and within days of starting them, you will feel better and have more confidence.

Just as brushing your teeth for a few minutes each day takes care of your dental health for life, these quick everyday habits will help move you towards sustainable weight loss. I would love you to get to the stage where you are effortlessly doing all three every day, but feel free to start with one and build up slowly. Remember, each of them takes under 5 minutes to do!

Doing these small habits consistently sends your body a powerful daily signal that you are worth taking care of. Don't be fooled by their ease—they're incredibly effective when done consistently. Once you have them ingrained into your daily life, it will make it much easier to implement the other ideas and principles in the book.

To increase your chances of success, stick these new habits onto a behavior you already do automatically and as part of your daily routine, e.g., boiling the kettle, making a coffee, your commute into work, or just before bed. Spend some time experimenting with the best time in your day for each one.

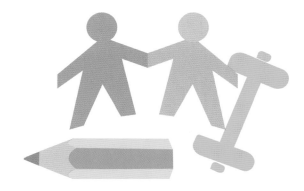

1 LIFT

Lift something every day. (page 146)

Keep a dumb-bell or kettlebell in your kitchen. When you go in there each morning to make a hot drink or for breakfast, lift it. Even if all you do is five bicep curls, you're showing your body each day that you're a thriving human. When you've finished, make sure you allow yourself to feel good about it. Start small, but try and build up to a five-minute workout (or more!) each morning, as I do. (See pages 148/149.)

2 CONNECT

Connect each day with another human being. (page 86–87)

I often see people soothing their loneliness with food. That is why each day, I want you to connect with another human being in a meaningful way. It doesn't need to take long. If you feel you don't have the connections for this, join a supportive online community. We'd all love to see you over at my Facebook group (https://www.facebook.com/groups/drchatterjeetribe/) (See page 233 for more ideas.)

3 REFLECT

Make time each day to see how far you've come. (page 111–12)

Many of us live our lives at a hundred miles an hour and we're often too busy to stop, think, and reflect. If you're going to change your relationship with your health in the long term, taking some time for yourself each day to reflect on how things are going is one of the most powerful things you can do. It needn't take long—even just a few minutes will suffice.

3 x BOOSTERS

These three boosters are additional areas that you may wish to spend some extra time on. They are not essential for everyone. However, many of my patients find them transformative and the key to unlocking their weight-loss journey.

You don't necessarily need to focus on these boosters right at the start of your plan, unless, of course, you identify them as a priority in the "Prepare Your Mind" exercise on page 247.

Even if you don't immediately feel they might be relevant for you, they are well worth experimenting with if you hit a plateau or roadblock.

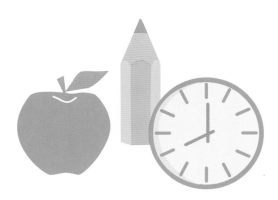

1 EMOTIONS AND STRESS

This is often the most important issue to address, as underlying, unresolved emotions or stress can often drive eating behavior.

- **The Freedom Exercise** (page 93)
- **The Five-Finger Breathing Technique** (page 96)
- **Fixing Your Self-Talk** (page 100)
- **Out of the Dark and Into the Light** (page 108)

2 FOOD TIMING

Some of my patients find changing when they eat is the secret to unlocking their weight-loss journey.

- **Limit Snacking** (page 167)
- **Eat Earlier in the Day** (page 171)
- **Take Control of Your Eating Window** (page 179)

3 PAYING ATTENTION TO WHAT WE EAT

When we pay attention to what and how we are eating, we often end up eating more in sync with what our bodies actually need.

- **Eat With Others, Not With Devices** (page 193)
- **Ten Minutes of Solitude** (page 194)
- **Make Cooking Time Fun** (page 197)
- **Eat Mindfully** (page 202)
- **A Mindful Moment of Bliss** (page 204)
- **Tell Your Body It's Time To Eat** (page 207)

YOUR LIFE, YOUR PLAN

Now you've looked around the toolbox, it's time for you to prioritize which areas you are going to start working on. On the page opposite, or on a fresh piece of paper, write down the specific actions that you are committing to for the week ahead. Stick it on the kitchen fridge or somewhere else highly visible. Try not to write too many actions down at once, as this can feel overwhelming.

Remember: everyone's plan will look different. Some of you will only feel ready to commit to one everyday habit at the start. Others, however, will want to commit to all three everyday habits *and* start work on all three foundations. Some of you will feel that your emotions are the priority and may wish to spend some time with the Freedom Exercise along with some of the everyday habits. And someone else who struggles with their sleep may choose to mostly focus on actions in that area. It doesn't really matter *where* or *how* you start. As long as you start.

Be really specific with your actions. For example, if you are working on your sleep—don't just write down "Prioritize Sleep." Instead, write down the specific things that you are committing to do, e.g., no caffeine after noon, 20 minutes of natural light every morning, no technology for 1 hour before bed.

Aim to re-evaluate your plan on a weekly basis (perhaps on a Sunday) to assess what has worked well and what needs changing. It may be you have a busy week ahead and need to reduce how many actions you are committing to, or it could be that you have transformed your sleep and no longer need to focus on that area and, instead, can turn your attention elsewhere.

Ideas and inspiration alone will not lead to change. Only taking action will do that. Write down your actions, commit to them, and watch your life change.

MY COMMITMENT TO MYSELF—THIS WEEK I WILL:

Once you have written your actions down, share them on social media using #feelgreatloseweight—this will not only help to keep you motivated, it will also encourage your friends to do and share their own, which in turn will help create your very own supportive healthy living tribe.

A TOOLBOX FOR LIFE

Use my recommendations above as a guide only. Feel free to modify and tweak them according to your needs and your life. Remember: I want you to be in charge.

I would recommend that you don't use scales as your daily barometer of success. In my experience, they can risk sabotaging your progress (see page 224). We often become far too attached to the number they flash up and this can lead to a roller coaster of different emotions, from euphoric joy to hopeless despair.

Instead, throughout your journey, focus on how you feel. In your daily reflection (one of your everyday habits), notice the increases in your energy and confidence and the improvements in your mood. These are the factors that will keep you going when your motivation starts to wane. If you really can't manage without your scales, try looking at them no more than once or twice a month.

As you go beyond the initial few weeks, remember to be kind to yourself. Sometimes, life gets stressful and we revert to old habits. That is completely okay. When this does happen, make sure you take some time to reflect and understand why. This is another opportunity to learn.

Whenever you hit a plateau, I would encourage you to revisit the "Preparation" section on page 246. It is amazing how often little things in our environment creep back in and start to influence our choices and how our priorities can change over time. A few days spent here can prove invaluable.

If, at any point, you feel particularly busy, take the pressure off yourself. This is not an all-or-nothing plan; it has been designed to work alongside the rest of your life. You cannot "fail" the plan by having a few bad days. If and when you feel stressed and busy, try focussing solely on the three everyday habits, even if all you manage is one of them. That one habit is still you doing something proactive for your health each day, and that is the secret to long-term success.

You will lose weight. It may not be as quick as you would like. It may not be as quick as your friend, who bought the latest "drop a dress size in two weeks" book. But it will be longer lasting, sustainable, and, most importantly, enjoyable along the way.

And if your friends ask you what "plan" you are following, you can tell them that you no longer follow other people's plans—because, you have been empowered to create your own.

Be patient. This will work but, like all good things in life, it takes time.

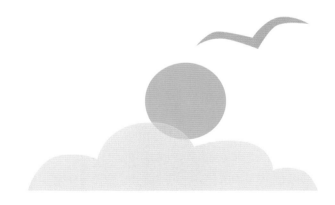

CONCLUSION

There's more to weight loss than you've been led to believe. The good news is that reaching a healthy size and staying there isn't a matter of starving yourself in the kitchen and hitting the gym hard. Any lifestyle program that makes you feel terrible is going to have terrible results. The fact is, rapid weight loss isn't really weight loss at all. It's an illusion. It doesn't last and, worse, it raises your weight point, meaning you'll probably end up with a bigger problem than you started with.

Keeping it off for good means losing weight and feeling great. It's a longer process, but it's much more fun. You'll be learning about yourself, understanding your behaviors and nourishing your body and mind with nutritious food and positive thoughts. Over time, you'll feel happier, less stressed, and more energetic, and the excess fat will start to naturally disappear.

Remember: you're not going for perfect. It would be nearly impossible to commit to every page of this book fully. You're looking for enough. This means regular small steps in the right direction. Don't worry if you have a bad day. Each morning, the sun rises again and that's a brand-new opportunity to make different choices. Throw away the scales and start focussing on those little daily habits that will add up to huge changes.

And don't wait. Too many of my patients have some golden future in their minds when they're at some ideal weight; they make the mistake of putting their life and happiness on hold until they get there. But your life is happening now. Your today is just as important as your tomorrow, your next month, and your next year. You can begin the journey of nourishing yourself, mind, heart, and body, the moment you put this book down.

It's time. Not just to live, but to live greatly.

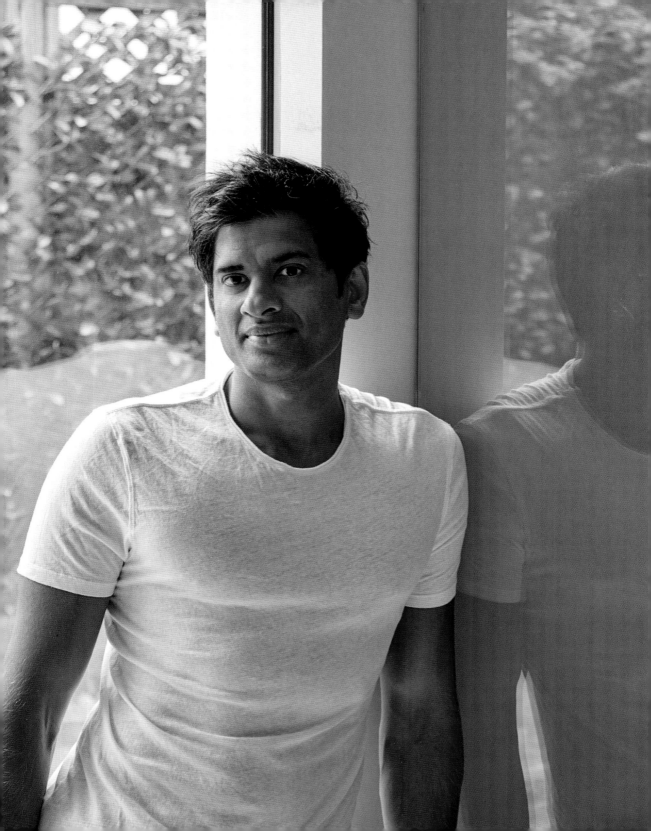

SOURCES AND FURTHER READING

SOURCES

1. WHAT WE EAT

K. D. Hall et al., "Ultra-processed Diets Cause Excess Calorie Intake and Weight Gain: An Inpatient Randomized Controlled Trial of *ad libitum* Food Intake," *Clinical and Translational Report*, 30(1), May 2019: 67–77, https://doi.org/10.1016/j.cmet.2019.05.008

L. S. Roe, J. S. Meengs and B. J. Rolls, "Salad and Satiety: The Effect of Timing of Salad Consumption on Meal Energy Intake," *Appetite*, 58(1), February 2012, 242–8, https://www.ncbi.nlm.nih.gov/pubmed/22008705

N. Wright et al., "The BROAD Study: A Randomised Controlled Trial Using a Whole Food Plant-based Diet in the Community for Obesity, Ischaemic Heart Disease or Diabetes," *Nutrition & Diabetes*, 7, March 2017, https://www.nature.com/articles/nutd20173

2. WHY WE EAT

Eating Your Emotions

P. Christiansen et al., "Alcohol's Acute Effect on Food is Mediated by Inhibitory Control Impairments," *Health Psychology*, 35(5), May 2016, 518–22, https://www.ncbi.nlm.nih.gov/pubmed/26690634

C. K. Ip et al., "Amygdala NPY Circuits Promote the Development of Accelerated Obesity under Chronic Stress Conditions," *Cell Metabolism*, 30(1), April 2019, 111–28, http://dx.doi.org/10.1016/j.cmet.2019.04.001

V. J. Felitti et al., "Relationship of Childhood Abuse and Household Dysfunction to Many of the Leading Causes of Death in Adults: The Adverse Childhood Experiences (ACE) Study," *American Journal of Preventive Medicine*, 14(4), May 1998: 245–258, https://www.ajpmonline.org/article/S0749-3797(98)00017-8/abstract

American Psychological Association report, 2007, https://www.apa.org/news/press/releases/2007/10/stress

Prioritize Sleep

L. Brondel et al., "Acute Partial Sleep Deprivation Increases Food Intake in Healthy Men," *American Journal of Clinical Nutrition*, 91(6), June 2010, 1550–59, https://pubmed.ncbi.nlm.nih.gov/20357041/

A-M. Chang et al., "Evening Use of Light-emitting eReaders Negatively Affects Sleep, Circadian Timing, and Next-Morning Alertness," *Proceedings of the National Academy of Sciences of the United States of America*, 112(4), December 2014, https://www.pnas.org/content/112/4/1232

K. V. Danilenko, S. V. Mustafina and E. A. Pechenkina, "Bright Light for Weight Loss: Results of a Controlled Crossover Trial," *Obes* Facts, 6(1), February 2013, 28–38, https://pubmed.ncbi.nlm.nih.gov/23429094/

K. J. Reid et al., "Timing and Intensity of Light Correlate with Body Weight in Adults," *PLoS One*, 9(4), April 2014, https://journals.plos.org/plosone/article?id=10.1371/journal.pone.0092251

M-P. St-Onge et al., "Short Sleep Duration Increases Energy Intake but Does Not Change Energy Expenditure in Normal-weight Individuals," *American Journal of Clinical Nutrition*, 94(2), August 2011, 410–16, https://academic.oup.com/ajcn/article/94/2/410/4597826

K. Spiegel et al., "Brief Communication: Sleep Curtailment in Healthy Young Men is Associated with Decreased Leptin Levels, Elevated Grehlin Levels, and Increased Hunger and Appetite", *Annals of Internal Medicine*, 141(11), December 2004, 846–50, https://pubmed.ncbi.nlm.nih.gov/15583226/

B. Wood et al., "Light Level and Duration of Exposure Determine the Impact of Self-luminous Tablets on Melatonin Suppression," *Applied Ergonomica*, 44(2), March 2013, 237–40, https://www.ncbi.nlm.nih.gov/pubmed/22850476

Move to Feel Alive

A. Jenkinson, *Why We Eat (Too Much)*, Penguin Random House UK, 2020

H. Pontzer et al., "Constrained Total Energy Expenditure and Metabolic Adaption to Physical Activity in Adult Humans," *Current Biology*, 26, February 2016, 410–17, https://www.cell.com/current-biology/pdf/S0960-9822(15)01577-8.pdf

H. Pontzer et al., "Hunter-gatherer Energetics and Human Obesity," *PLoS ONE*, July 2012, https://journals.plos.org/plosone/article?id=10.1371/journal.pone.0040503

S. Guyenet, *The Hungry Brain*, Vermillion, 2017

3. WHEN YOU EAT

M. Garaulet et al., "Timing of Food Intake Predicts Weight Loss Effectiveness," *International Journal of Obesity*, 37, January 2013, 604–11, https://www.nature.com/articles/ijo2012229

D. Jakubowicz et al., "High Caloric Intake at Breakfast vs. Dinner Differentially Influences Weight Loss of Overweight and Obese Women," *Obesity*, 21(12), March 2013, https://onlinelibrary.wiley.com/doi/full/10.1002/oby.20460

H. Kahleova et al., "Eating Two Larger Meals a Day (Breakfast and Lunch) is More Effective than Six Smaller Meals in a Reduced-energy Regimen for Patients with Type 2 Diabetes: A Randomised Crossover Study," *Diabetologia,* 57(8), May 2014, 1551–60, https://www.ncbi.nlm.nih.gov/pmc/articles/PMC4079942/

M. Lombardo et al., "Morning Meal More Efficient for Fat Loss in a 3-month Lifestyle Intervention," *Journal of the American College of Nutrition*, 33(3), May 2014, 198–205, https://pubmed.ncbi.nlm.nih.gov/24809437/

W. McHill et al., "Later Circadian Timing of Food Intake is Associated with Increased Body Fat," *American Journal of Clinical Nutrition*, 106(5), November 2017, 1213–19, https://academic.oup.com/ajcn/article/106/5/1213/4822338?sid=0b186230-db4a-42ea-a0f8-a5efd1945432

T. Moro et al., "Effects of Eight Weeks of Time-restricted Feeding (16/8) on Basal Metabolism, Maximal Strength, Body Composition, Inflammation, and Cardiovascular Risk Factors in Resistance-trained Males," *Journal of Translational Medicine*, 290, 2016, https://doi.org/10.1186/s12967-016-1044-0

4. HOW WE EAT

E. Robinson et al., "Eating Attentively: A Systematic Review and Meta-analysis of the Effect of Food Intake Memory and Awareness on Eating," *American Journal of Clinical Nutrition*, 97(4), April 2013, 728–42, https://academic.oup.com/ajcn/article/97/4/728/4577025

R. I. M. Dunbar, "Breaking Bread: the Functions of Social Eating," *Adaptive Human Behavior and Physiology*, 3, March 2017: 198–211, https://link.springer.com/article/10.1007/s40750-017-0061-4

5. WHERE WE EAT

D. Buettner and S. Skemp, "Blue Zones: Lessons from the World's Longest Lived," *American Journal of Lifestyle Medicine*, 10(5), Sept–Oct 2016, https://www.ncbi.nlm.nih.gov/pmc/articles/PMC6125071/

N. Christakis, "The Hidden Influence of Social Networks," *TED*, 2010, https://www.ted.com/talks/nicholas_christakis_the_hidden_influence_of_social_networks/transcript?language=en

N. A. Christakis and J. H. Fowler, "The Spread of Obesity in a Large Social Network over 32 Years," *New England Journal of Medicine*, 357, July 2007, 370–79, http://www.nejm.org/doi/full/10.1056/NEJMsa066082

FURTHER READING

B. J. Fogg, *Tiny Habits: The Small Changes that Change Everything*, Virgin Books, 2019

S. Guyenet, *The Hungry Brain: Outsmarting the Instincts that Make Us Overeat*, Vermilion, April 2017.

A. Jenkinson, *Why We Eat (Too Much)*, Penguin Random House UK, 2020

S. Panda, *The Circadian Code: Lose Weight, Supercharge Your Energy, and Transform Your Health from Morning to Midnight*, Vermilion, 2018

INDEX

ACKNOWLEDGMENTS

A few years ago, the idea of writing a book was nothing but a dream. Now, I sit in front of my fourth completed manuscript, with an overwhelming feeling of gratitude. I truly believe in the power of books. Much of what we consume these days is transient and short lived, but books are evergreen. Books become a part of people's lives in truly unique ways. In this fast-paced digital world, books are a reminder that we as humans are analogue beings. You can hold books in your hands, hear the pages as you turn them and, when you are done, put them on a shelf where they sit ready and primed for you to open again, when the need arises.

Contrary to what many people think, writing a book is not a solo pursuit—it requires the help of many. I am blessed to have a supportive family, incredible friends, remarkable colleagues, and a unique publisher in Penguin Life, who all believe in my mission. For this, I am truly grateful.

I've always felt that we can learn something from every single person we meet. So, in that way, every single person I have ever met in person or interacted with online has in some way influenced my thinking. However, there are a few people who I would like to give a special mention to:

To my patients—thank you. Over the past two decades you have shared your struggles and challenges with me and have helped me better understand the true causes of ill health. I am eternally grateful.

To my incredible wife, Vidhaata. You never cease to amaze me. You help guide me through life with your unwavering integrity and strong moral compass and you constantly challenge me to be the best I can be. Thank you for walking alongside me.

To Jainam and Anoushka, to whom this book is dedicated. Being with you both makes my heart sing. You light up my soul in ways that no one else can. You deserve to grow up in a world full of love, compassion, and kindness. Together, let's be the change we want to see in the world.

To Mum, Dad, and Dada—thanks for always providing a supportive environment for me to pursue my dreams.

To Chetana and Dinesh, you are both incredibly special people—I continue to learn so much from you both and your outlook on life.

To Tommy Wood—you have a voice that I have always resonated with. You have unrivalled expertise but what I value the most is your compassionate manner and your heartfelt desire to help people improve their health and lives. Thanks for proof-reading my manuscript—this book is better because of your input.

To my friends—I honestly feel I have the best group of friends anyone could wish for. I just wish you all lived closer to me! Jeremy, Ayan, Steve, Luke, Carron, Phil, Dhru, Jodie, Bobby, Ashley, Mark, Claire, Mike, and Antony—thank you for always having my back.

To Will Storr, you have been legendary, as always.

To Will Francis, I couldn't imagine writing a book without you in my corner. I am lucky to have you representing me.

To Clare Moore, I know I can always rely on you. Thank you for being there.

To Gareth Bowler—getting to know you over the past year has been one of the highlights. You are an incredible person with unique insights. Thanks for all that you do.

To Sophie Williams—thanks for all the work you do in helping me spread my message.

To Gary Ward, James Largey, B.J. Fogg, Brian Mackenzie, Andy Ramage—thanks for your professional input.

To Miranda Harvey, working with you again has been such a wonderful experience. You have shown incredible dedication to help bring the ideas in this book to life and have indulged me countless times in trying to make my last-minute ideas work! Your brilliant insights will result in many more people connecting with the content inside.

To Clare Winfield—you make photography look easy! Working with you is so much fun—not only because of the brilliant photos you take but also because of your warm and friendly manner—looking forward to the next time already.

Thanks also to Polly Webb-Wilson, Megan Davies and Chris Terry, as well as Kirsty, Zoe and Ellis at Janklow.

And last but not least, to the team of incredible women that I get to work with at Penguin Life: Venetia, Emily, Julia, Alice, Emma, Saffron, Amy—thank you for taking the time to truly understand my goals and helping me reach them.

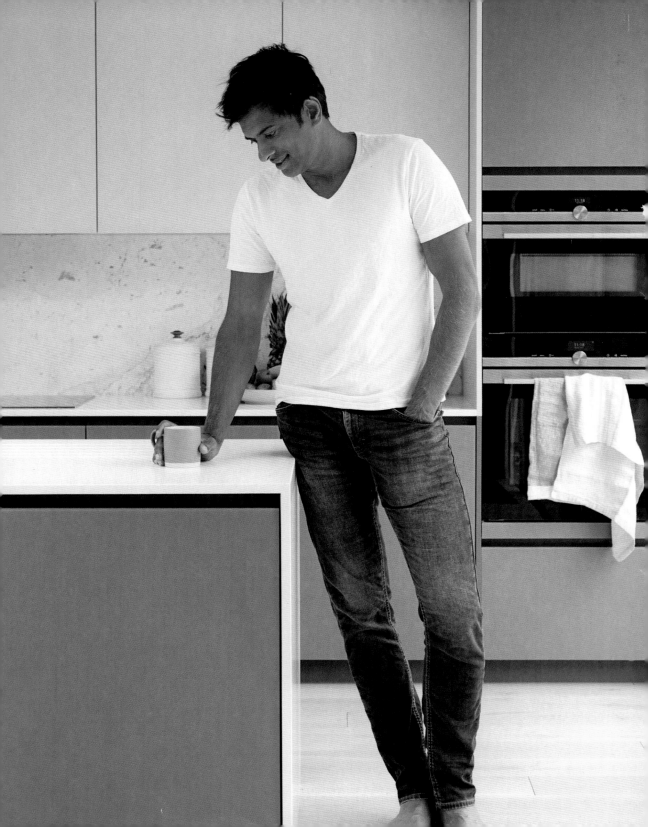